# A-Z OF HORSE DISEASES & HEALTH PROBLEMS

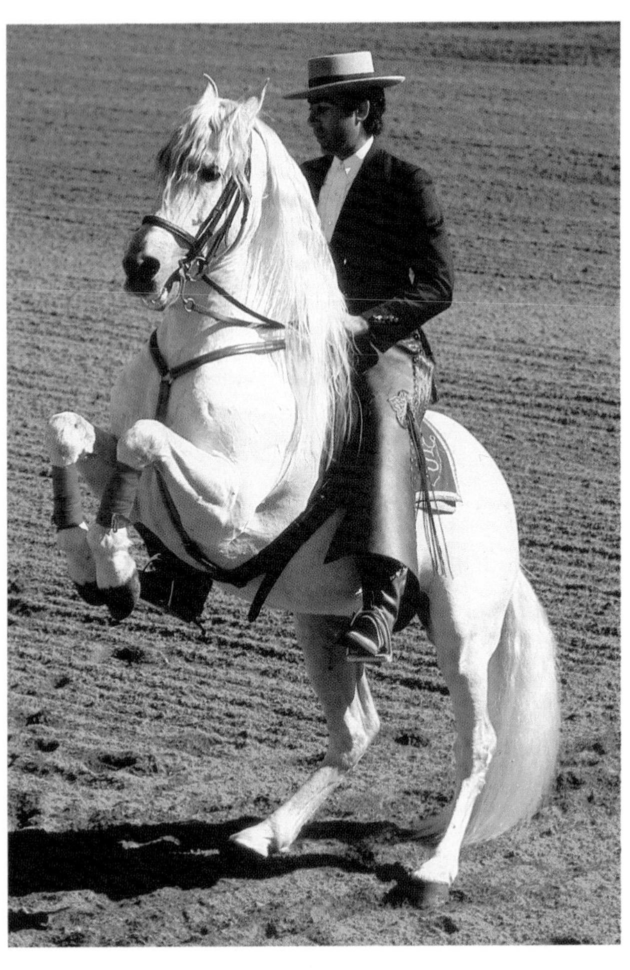

# A-Z OF HORSE DISEASES & HEALTH PROBLEMS

Signs • Diagnoses • Causes
Treatment

**Tim Hawcroft**
B.V.Sc (Hons), M.A.C.V.Sc.

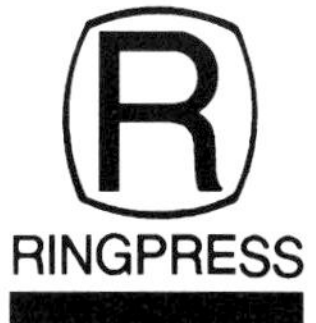

# ACKNOWLEDGMENTS

*Photographs:* Australian Jockey Club, 26, 122, 123; Vicki Cannon 59; Dr Neil Cooper, Bayer Veterinary Pharmaceutical Co 249, 250; Ethnor Pharmaceutical Co 251, 252, 253, 254; Dr W Hartley 55; Martin Hawcroft 77, 248; Bonny Lestikow 53, 60, 80, 206, 207, 208, 209, 210; Dr Derek Major 32, 33, 35, 72, 74, 75, 76, 92, 95, 119, 120, 130, 142, 180, 275, 299; S Neville 6; Pfizer Veterinary Pharmaceutical Co 42, 141, 181, 257; Prof Reuben Rose, University of Sydney 52, 59, 78, 96, 102, 126, 164, 231, 235; Dr J Smith 70, 71, 182, 188; other photographs by Ray Joyce/Weldon Trannies.

*Diagrams:* Jan Hawcroft 10–11, 18, 220.

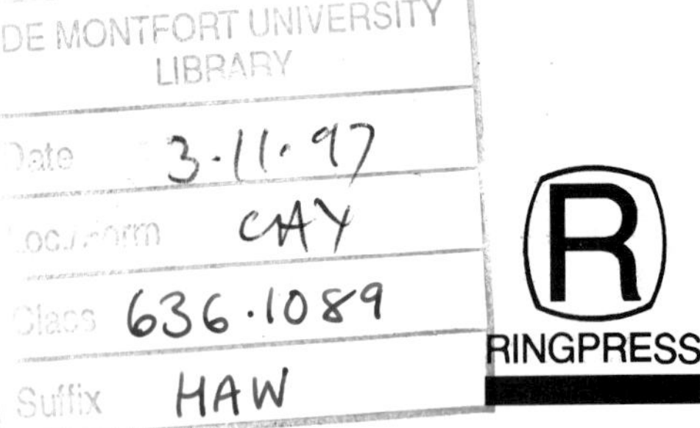




This edition published in the United Kingdom in 1993 by
Ringpress Books Limited
The Warren, Aylburton Common
Lydney, Gloucestershire GL15 6YD

Originated by Lansdowne Publishing Pty Ltd
Sydney, Australia

Reprinted 1994, 1995, 1997



Designed by Christie & Eckermann
Typset in Australia by Savage Type Pty Ltd, Brisbane
Printed in Singapore by Kyodo Printing Co. Pte Ltd

ISBN 0 948955 48 1

# CONTENTS

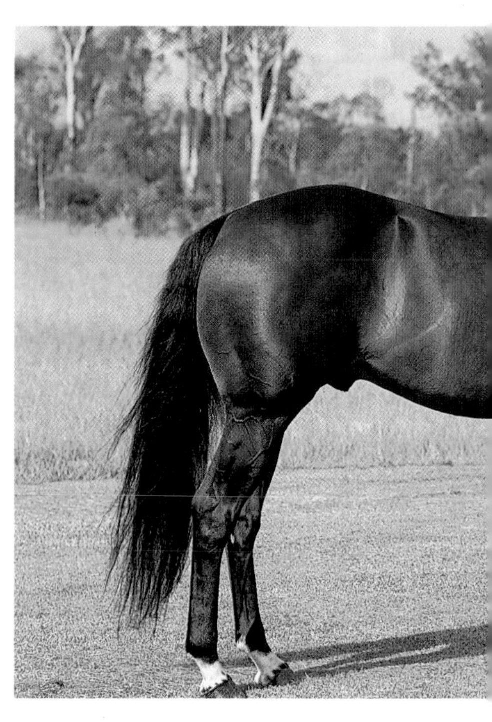

# INTRODUCTION

The numbers of breeders, stud masters, trainers, grooms, riders, owners, pony club members and horse lovers have increased greatly in recent years. All want to know more and more about the health of their horses. They are particularly concerned about being able to help a horse recover when it is distressed or not well. They are aware that they need ready access to information so that they can act quickly and with authority; so that they know when to call the veterinary surgeon, apply first aid, or begin the right treatment; so that they can manage an outbreak of disease or prevent it from spreading.

It is well to remember that the treatment of a health problem or disease in its early stages may bring about a quick recovery, relieve the horse of further pain and suffering, prevent it from becoming permanently disabled (unsound) and save its life.

Many equine diseases and health problems are set out in books in technical terms which the reader doesn't understand or remember. In trying to find out what is really wrong with a horse the reader has to search through

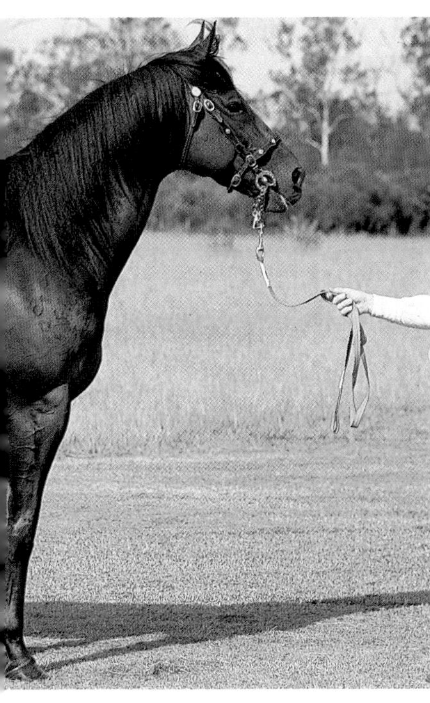

A healthy horse — well muscled and with a shiny coat

a lot of material, a time-consuming and often confusing exercise.

To remedy this situation, this guidebook has been written solely about the diseases and health problems of horses and the material in it structured so that the relevant information can be easily found. The book can be used on the spot, simply and quickly, by novice or expert, without prior knowledge of technical terminology.

Students and graduates of veterinary science, of horse care courses, of stud management and horse training programs, who are about to embark on their careers, will find the *A-Z of Horse Diseases and Health Problems* a supportive resource book. Amply illustrated and essentially practical, it is an excellent back-up book in decision making.

In the preparation of this book I would like to thank my wife Jan for her patient assistance, my children Melanie, Samantha, Damien and Edwina for their understanding of a father busy elsewhere, my father Eric for his ready assistance and advice and for preparing the index, my sister Judy for her helpful support and for typing the manuscript, and friends and colleagues for their encouragement.

*Tim Hawcroft*

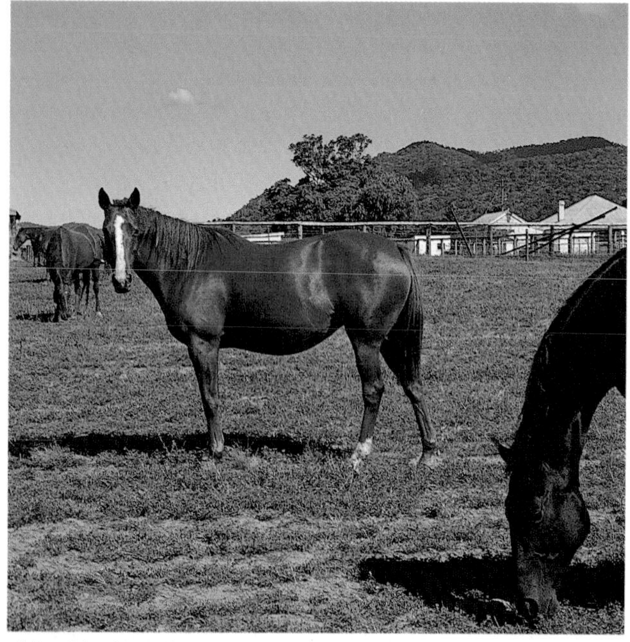

A healthy brood mare — note the shiny coat

# HOW TO USE THIS BOOK

The book begins with five short sections of information that will help you to care for your horse more effectively. The skeletal system and points of a horse are described to enable you to understand certain terms used in the book. The signs of a healthy horse are given in detail to provide you with a standard for evaluating the health status of a horse. When to call the veterinarian, practical hints for first aid, and how to administer medication complete this background information.

The two main sections of the book are:

**1 Signs of Diseases and Health Problems A–Z**

This section is concerned with helping you to recognise the signs and to diagnose what is wrong with your horse.

The best way of using this section is to take the book with you when observing your horse. Before beginning your observation it is a good idea to glance down the index of first signs (page 48) to get a general idea of what you are looking for.

When you have identified the first sign of your horse's disease or problem, turn to the page reference given in the index of first signs.

Here you will find your first sign linked with groups of associated signs, each with a possible diagnosis and page reference.

If you are in doubt about your possible diagnosis, return to the horse with this book and check as many signs as possible — or seek the advice of your veterinarian.

**2 Treatment of Diseases and Health Problems A–Z**

This section provides details of the signs, causes and treatment of the diseases and health problems diagnosed with the help of the section described above, Signs of Diseases and Health Problems A–Z.

Some treatments can be administered by a lay person but others should be left to the veterinarian.

# SKELETAL SYSTEM

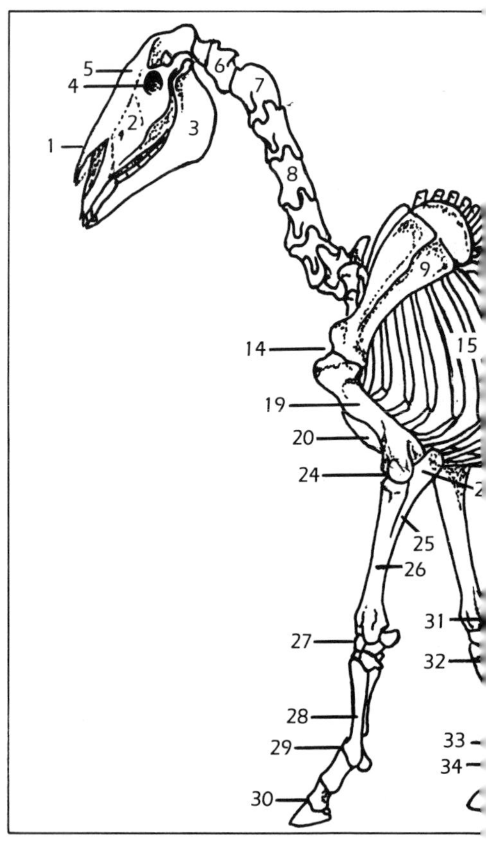


| | | | |
|---|---|---|---|
| 1 | Nasal bone | 12 | Sacral vertebrae |
| 2 | Maxillary bone | 13 | Coccygeal vertebrae |
| 3 | Mandible | 14 | Shoulder joint |
| 4 | Orbit | 15 | Ribs — 18 in number |
| 5 | Frontal bone | 16 | Pelvis |
| 6 | Atlas | 17 | Hip joint |
| 7 | Axis | 18 | Femur |
| 8 | Cervical vertebrae | 19 | Humerus |
| 9 | Scapula | 20 | Sternum |
| 10 | Thoracic vertebrae | 21 | Olecranon |
| 11 | Lumbar vertebrae | 22 | Stifle joint |

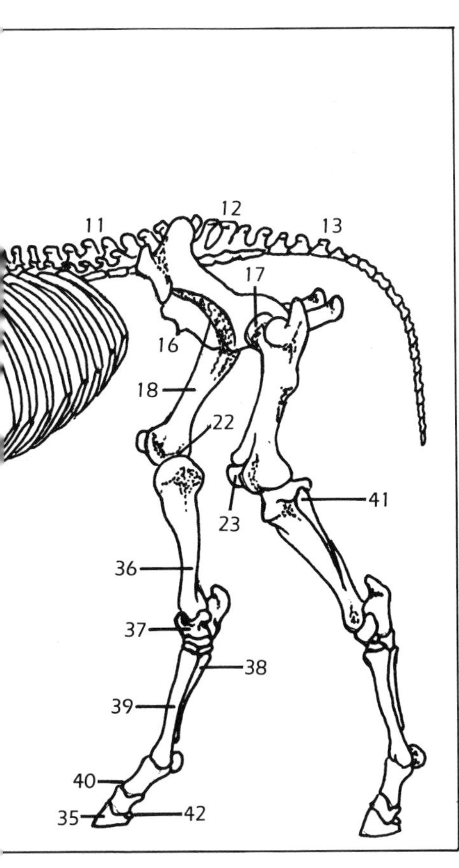


| | | | |
|---|---|---|---|
| 23 | Patella | 33 | Sesamoid bone |
| 24 | Elbow joint | 34 | First phalanx |
| 25 | Ulna | 35 | Pedal bone |
| 26 | Radius | 36 | Tibia |
| 27 | Carpus | 37 | Tarsal bones |
| 28 | Cannon (metacarpal) bone | 38 | Splint bone |
| 29 | Fetlock joint | 39 | Cannon bone |
| 30 | Coffin joint | 40 | Pastern joint |
| 31 | Accessory carpal bone | 41 | Fibula |
| 32 | Splint bone | 42 | Navicular bone |

# POINTS OF A HORSE

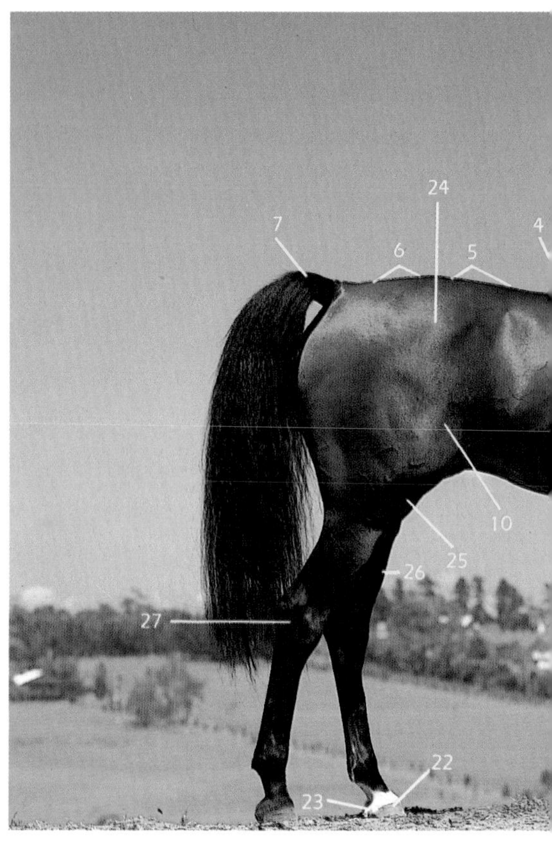


1 The poll is the bony prominence lying between the ears. Except for the ears, it is the highest point on the horse's body when it is standing with its head up.

2 The forelock is the hair that covers the forehead and grows from the poll area. It must not be confused with the fetlock.

3 The withers is the prominent ridge where the neck and back join. At this ridge, powerful muscles of the neck and shoulder attach to elongated spines of the second to the sixth thoracic vertebrae. The height of a horse is measured vertically from the withers to the ground, because the withers is the horse's highest constant point.

4 The back extends from the base of the withers to where the last rib is attached.

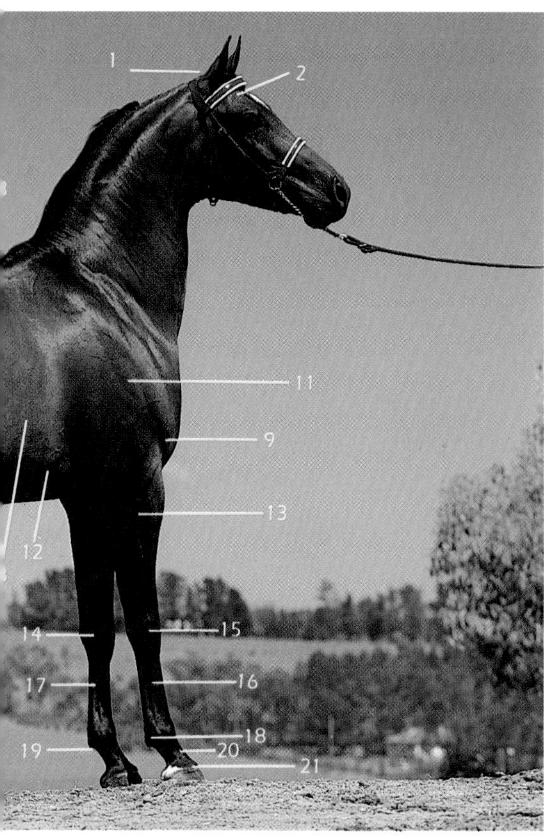


5 The loin or coupling is the short area joining the back to the powerful muscular croup (rump).

6 The croup (rump) lies between the loin and the tail. When one is looking from the side or back, it is the highest point of the hindquarters.

7 The dock is the bony portion of the tail that tapers to a point about one-third of the way down the tail.

8 The chest is encased by the ribs, extending from between the forelegs to the flanks.

9 The breast is a muscle mass between the forelegs, covering the front of the chest.

10 The flank is the area below the loin, between the last rib and the massive muscles of the thigh.

11 The point of the shoulder is a hard, bony prominence surrounded by heavy muscle masses. It is approximately level with the intersection of the lower line of the neck and the body.

12 The elbow is a bony prominence lying against the chest at the beginning of the forearm.

13 The forearm extends from the elbow to the knee.

14 The chestnuts are horny growths on the insides of the legs, located approximately halfway down.

15 The knee is the joint between the forearm and the cannon bone.

16 The cannon bone or shin, as it is called when in the foreleg, lies between the knee and the fetlock, and is visible from the front.

17 The flexor tendons run from the knee to the fetlock and can be seen lying behind the cannon bone.

18 The fetlock is the joint between the cannon bone and the pastern.

19 The ergot is a horny growth at the back of the fetlock, hidden by a tuft of hair.

20 The pastern extends from the fetlock to the top of the hoof (coronet).

21 The coronet is a band around the top of the hoof from which the hoof wall grows.

22 The hoof refers to the horny wall and sole of the foot. The foot includes the horny structure and the pedal and navicular bones, as well as other connective tissues.

23 The heels are the bulbs at the back of the hoof and, while horny in texture, they are softer than the normal hoof wall.

24 The point of the hip is a bony prominence lying just forward and below the croup. This is not the hip joint.

25 The stifle is a joint at the end of the thigh corresponding to the human knee.

26 The gaskin is the region between the stifle and the hock.

27 The hock is the joint between the gaskin and the cannon bone. The bony protuberance at the back is called the point of the hock. It may be easily injured, especially when the horse kicks.

# SIGNS OF A HEALTHY HORSE

## Appetite

Some horses are fussy about their feed. Familiarise yourself with the type and volume of feed they like and each morning and evening check the feed bin to see how much has been eaten. If little or none, check the palatability of the feed and whether or not there has been any change in quality or type. If there is no logical explanation for loss of appetite, regard it as one of the first signs of illness.

## Coat and skin

Coat will vary with breed, season and housing conditions (stabled and/or rugged). For instance, the thoroughbred has a fine coat in summer; the shetland pony has a long, thick, two-layered coat in winter. Whether the coat is long or short, thick or fine, it should be evenly distributed except during the process of shedding the winter coat in spring. Normally, the coat should be soft with a lustre. The skin should be supple and elastic with no sign of bald patches, rubbing, inflammation or ooze.

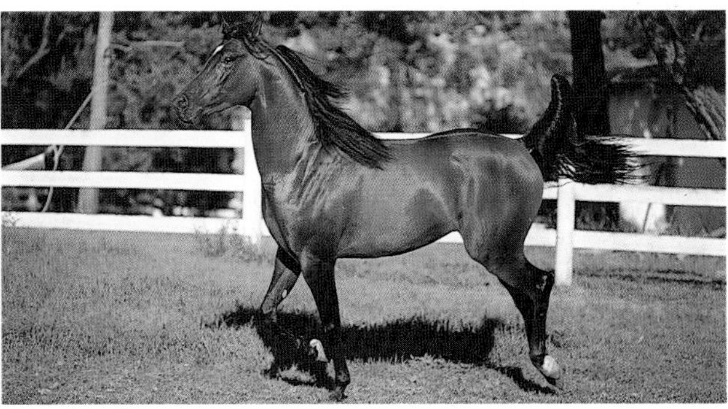

A healthy horse

## Condition (weight)

A horse's condition varies with breeds, feed and exercise. Condition can also vary within breeds; some may be in well-muscled condition, others may be fat or thin. A thin horse is not necessarily unhealthy. A horse on the same ration and exercise routine maintains a certain weight for years. If suddenly, or over a period of time, it starts to lose weight, check your horse carefully. Weight loss or gain in association with some other sign, e.g. poor coat, diarrhoea, poor appetite, lethargy or poor work peformance, is indicative of a health problem.

## Conformation

To examine a horse's conformation, look at it standing still from a short distance away to ascertain overall balance, then examine it more closely for body detail, limb detail and relationship of limbs to each other. The horse should then be observed in motion to evaluate its co-ordination.

### *Body conformation*

The relationship between the conformation of the body and limbs is more important than body conformation itself; the body should be well-proportioned and in balance with the limbs. Size varies between different breeds and should be taken into account when evaluating a horse. However, certain conformation characteristics such as angle and length of pastern are common to all breeds.

Horses with near-perfect conformation are rare. When buying a horse you have to weigh up the good points against the bad, taking into account the purpose for which the horse will be used. Don't lower your standards and always aim to purchase a horse with perfect conformation.

The head should be neither too big nor too small, well-set on the neck and intelligent looking. The forehead should be broad, with eyes set well apart, and the nostrils large with well-defined edges. The carriage of the head should not be too high or too low, or it will interfere with the horse's sight and balance. The neck can be a very attractive feature. It should be of ample length (i.e. in correct proportion to head and body) with an arch, curved top line and straight bottom line.

The muscles of the shoulders should be well-developed. A long sloping shoulder allows greater flexibility of joint, permitting a longer stride and giving a smoother ride; straight, upright shoulders can increase concussion and give a rough, unpleasant ride. The chest should be rounded and have plenty of depth (a good girth). The width of chest between the forelegs should be sufficient to eliminate any friction between the forelimbs.

Located at the base of the neck, the withers are the high point of a horse's back. From this point a horse's height is measured. Width, height and length of withers should be sufficient to provide good anchorage for the saddle; thin, over-prominent withers are prone to saddle damage.

The back should be strong because it bears the weight of the rider. Long backs are weaker than shorter ones and predispose the horse to back strain; short backs predispose the horse to interference between hind and front limbs

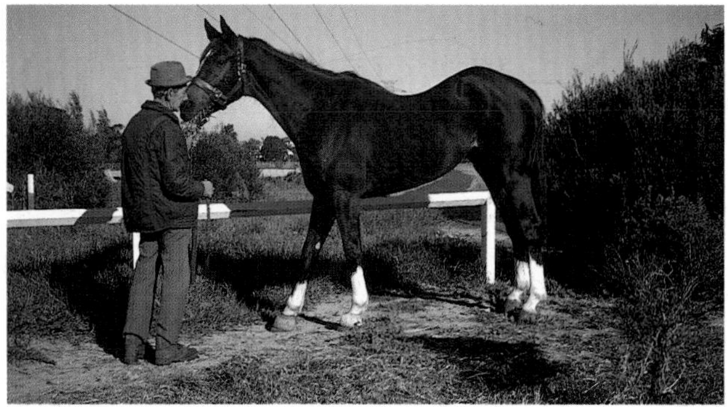

Sway back — the line of the back is too concave

when in motion. The line of back should not be too concave (sway back) nor in any way convex (roach back).

The quarters should be powerful (well-muscled) but in proportion with the rest of the body. From this region of the body, the horse gets most of its forward thrust when galloping and jumping. Top of the hindquarters should be rounded, i.e. not falling away too sharply.

## *Limb conformation*

**Forelimb** To assess, the horse should be standing squarely on a flat, hard surface, bearing its weight equally on all four legs. When the horse is seen from the front the chest should appear to be well-developed and well-muscled and the legs should be straight. An imaginary line drawn from point of shoulder to foot should divide the leg into two equal parts. Toes of feet should point straight forward and feet should be as wide apart on the ground as the origin of the legs at the chest. Knees should be flat, not deviating towards or away from each other. Cannon bone should be centred under the knee.

From the side, an imaginary vertical line from the spinous process of the shoulder blade should divide the leg into two equal parts down to the fetlock joint and continue to ground level to a point just behind the heel. Muscles of the forearm should be well-developed and should balance the limb. The knee should not bend forward (standing over at the knee) or backward (back at the knee). The cannon bone should not give the impression of being tied-in below the knee. The pastern should be of correct length, i.e. in proportion to the total length of the leg. The hoof wall should slope at the same angle as the pastern.

**Hind limb** When the horse is studied from behind, an imaginary vertical line drawn from the point of the pelvis

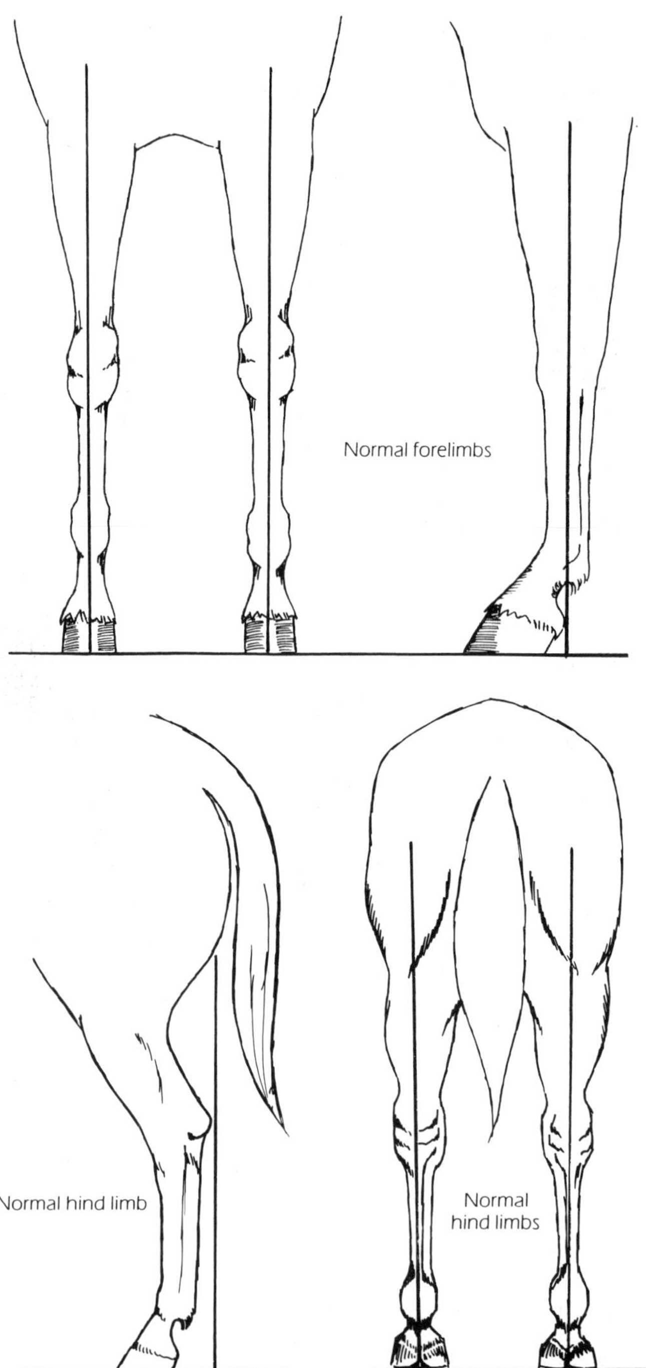
Normal forelimbs
Normal hind limb
Normal
hind limbs

should divide the leg into two equal parts. The hocks should be large, strong, clean and well-defined. When viewed from the side, a vertical line drawn from the point of the pelvis should touch the point of the hock, run down the rear aspect of the cannon bone and touch ground 7–10 cm behind the heels. The angle of stifle and hock should be neither too straight nor too acute.

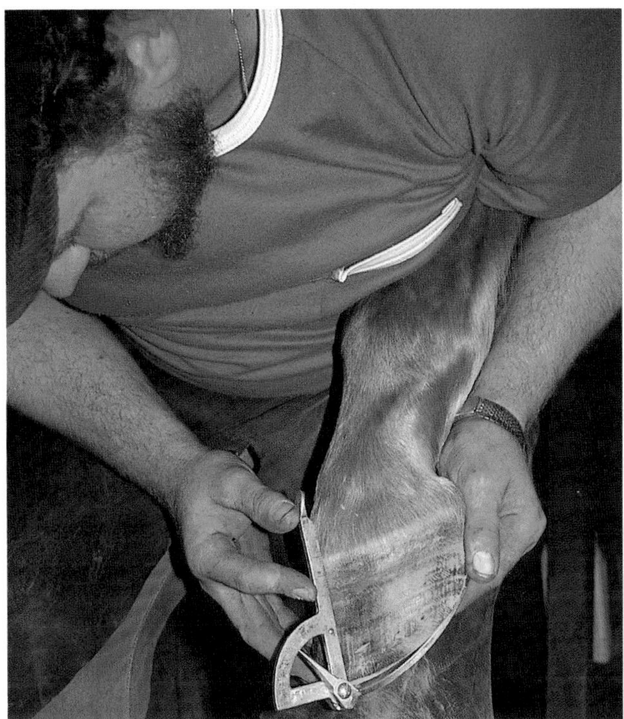

Checking the angle made by the hoof wall and the sole

The forefoot should be round at the toe and wide at the heels. The hoof wall should be thickest at the toe, thinning at quarter and thicker at heel. The sole should be moderately concave. Ideal angle made by the face of wall and sole at toe is 45–50 degrees. The frog, which divides the sole into halves, should be well-developed and rubbery in consistency; when the horse is bearing its weight on the foot, the frog should be touching the ground.

The hind foot is more pointed at the toe and its sole is more concave than that of the forefoot. The angle made by the face of the wall and sole at the toe of the hind foot is 50–55 degrees.

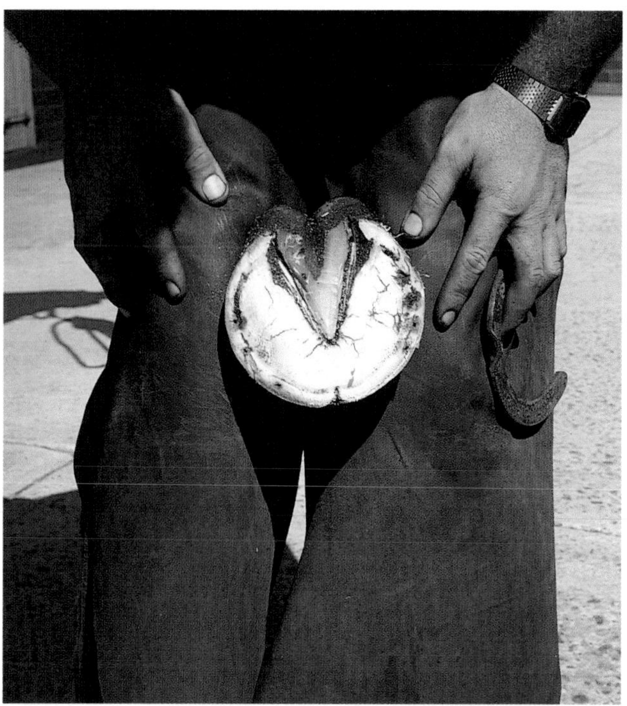

The frog divides the sole into halves

## Demeanour

This may vary tremendously in different breeds, individuals and situations. When approached, the horse's normal demeanour is to move away, stand or come to you. Moving away may present a problem of catching. Changes in demeanour such as quiet to excited, alert to dull, placid to aggressive, relaxed to restless may indicate a more significant problem.

## Droppings (manure)

This usually occurs 10–15 times a day. Colour, consistency, volume, odour and frequency of droppings vary considerably with type of feed and exercise. A horse on a well-balanced diet should pass droppings that are brown, formed, tend to break up as they hit the ground and have an odour that is not unpleasant. Horses on lush green feed will often pass greenish, unformed, cow-like droppings; those on large volumes of low-grade hay will pass hard, dark-coloured pellets.

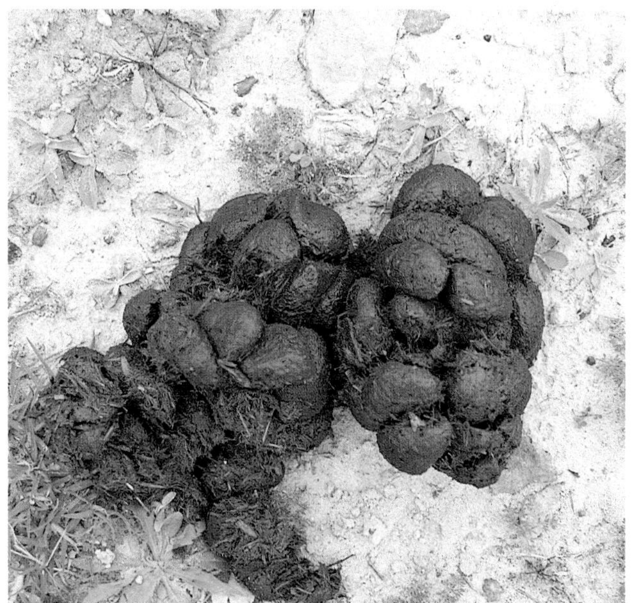

Normal droppings

## Ears

These should stand erect in an alert but not rigid position. One ear should not flop nor should there be any sign of discharge or heavy wax build-up.

## Eyes

The surface of the eye should be glistening, clear and moist, the conjunctiva glistening pink. The pupil should not be excessively dilated or constricted but will vary with light conditions. The eyeball should not be sunken or protrude and both eyeballs should be the same size. Eyelids should open without excessive blinking, the rim of the eyelid should be in contact with the eyeball, and the nictitating membrane (third eyelid) can be seen in corner of eye but not protruding to cover part of the eye. There should be no visible discharge, either clear or pus-coloured, from the eye.

## Gait

The ideal surface on which to see a horse walk and trot is a smooth, hard one such as bitumen. The feet should be studied as they leave the ground, during their flight through the air and as they land. Listening to the sound

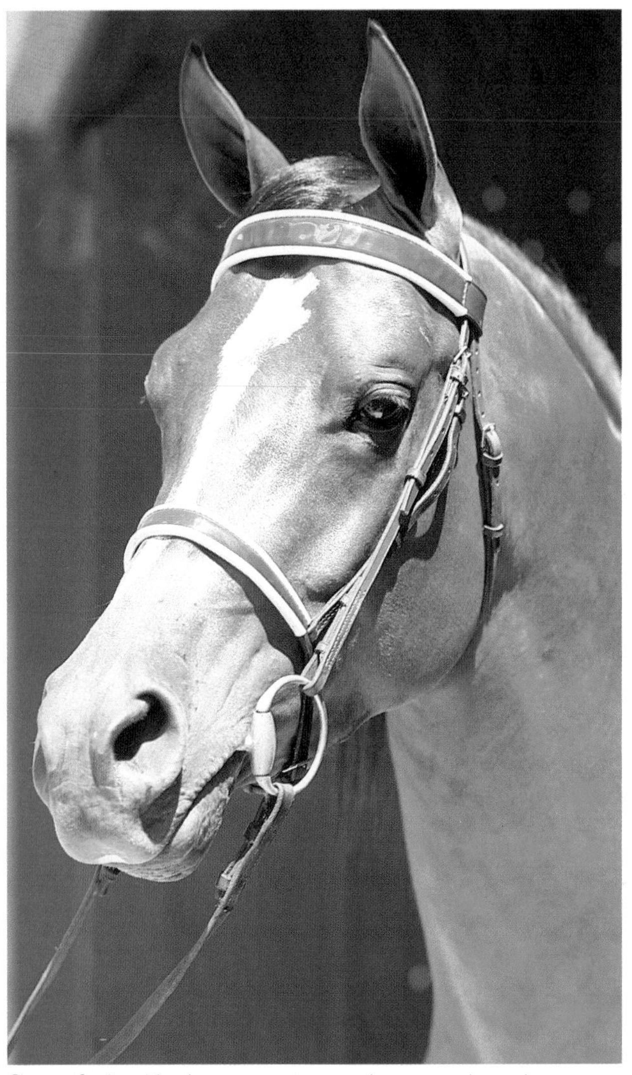

Signs of a healthy horse: erect ears, clear eye, clean dry mouth, clean open nostrils

of the feet as they land is a useful technique in evaluating rhythm of the gait.

The horse on a lead should be walked briskly in a straight line away from you for 50 metres, then turned and walked straight back towards you. As the horse approaches, step to one side and observe it from the side as it passes by. Carry out the same procedure with the horse at trot. In this situation you are watching to see if the limbs move in a straight line. Any deviation is wasted effort, increases the risk of one limb interfering with another and may place undue strain on a section of the limb. The stride should be long and free with a certain rhythm in the 'way of going' of all four legs. The horse should negotiate all turns freely; shuffling around them is undesirable and could indicate soreness or restricted flexibility in a joint.

You should also observe the horse's action, a term used to describe the amount of flexion of knees and hocks. Horses used for different purposes have different actions, e.g. the hackney has a high knee and hock action, the racehorse has a free-moving, long-striding, 'daisy cutting' action. Generally, the horse in moving should not have a proppy, stilted action, step short, or nod its head.

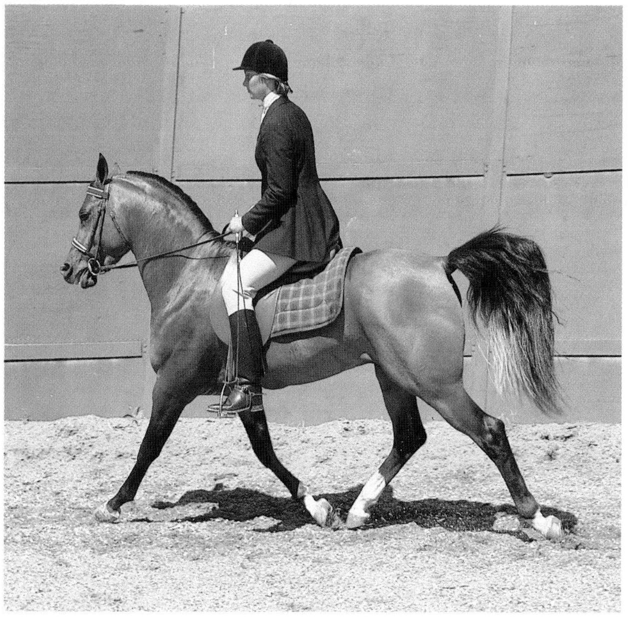

This horse has a good free action at the trot

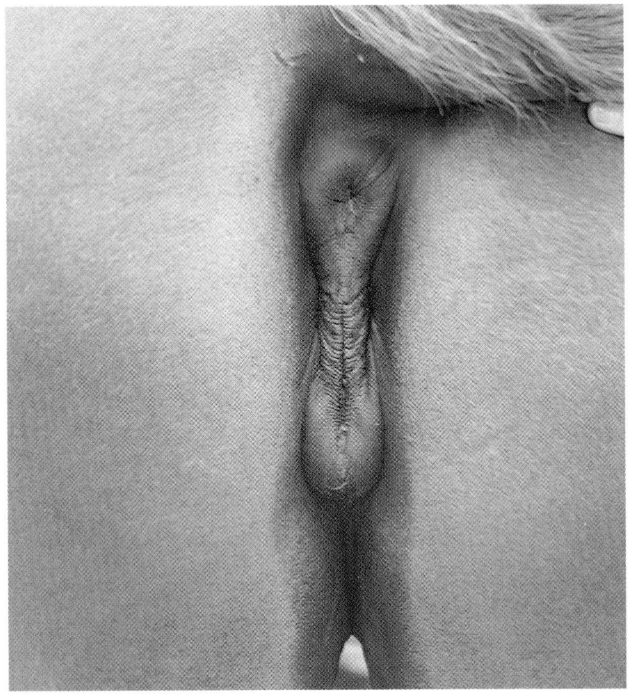

A normal vulva

## Genitalia

In the mare the lips of the vulva should oppose each other and there should be no sign of pus or blood from the vagina.

In the stallion or gelding, the prepuce (sheath) should not be swollen or show any pus discharge. The penis when seen during urination or sexual arousal will show signs of scale, waxy secretion and debris in folds unless cleaned regularly. A very small scrotum may indicate a testicle problem.

## Heart rate

The resting heart rate for a horse is 30–40 beats per minute with a regular rhythm. To detect, place palm of hand on chest behind point of elbow of near (left) foreleg positioned about one-third of a metre in front of off (right) leg.

## Mouth

Lips should be clean and dry. There should be no sign of excess saliva (stringy or frothy), pus, blood or unpleasant odour. Teeth should be regular and have no sharp edges.

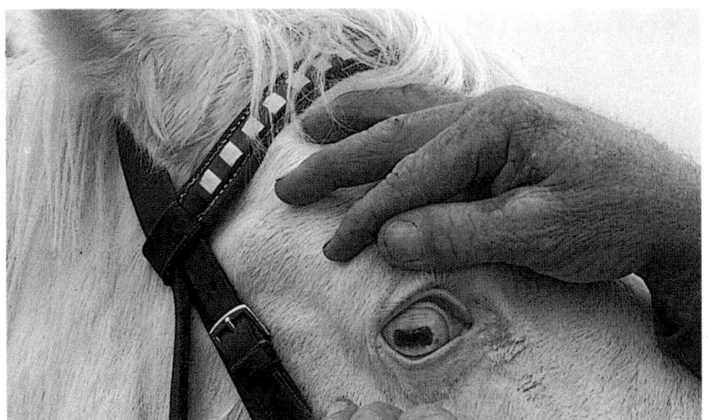

Healthy conjunctiva (the pink membrane around the eye)

## Mucous membranes

The usual ones to examine are the conjunctiva (membrane around eye) and gums. They should be deep pink in colour, not dark red (congested), bright red (inflamed), yellow (jaundice), pale or white (anaemic), or blue (cyanotic, i.e. lacking in oxygen). The membrane should be moist and glistening, not dry nor wet with excess secretion.

## Nostrils

Nostrils should be open, not unduly flared, clean and dry, and free from discharge. Air movement in and out of both nostrils should flow freely and there should be no unpleasant odour.

## Posture

Normal posture for the horse is standing. There are various ligaments and tendons in the forelimbs from the elbow down which lock the legs into a rigid rod when bearing weight equally on both front legs. They are referred to as the 'stay apparatus' which enables the horse to sleep and rest standing up.

Some horses lie down when in familiar, safe, comfortable surroundings. If the horse is lying down for lengthy periods of time or continues to lie down when approached, especially by a stranger, then something is wrong. If the horse is getting up and down, looking at its flanks, pawing the ground regularly, it indicates a problem.

## Respiration

Normal respiration rate is 10–15 breaths per minute. First examine the horse's respiration from a distance of about

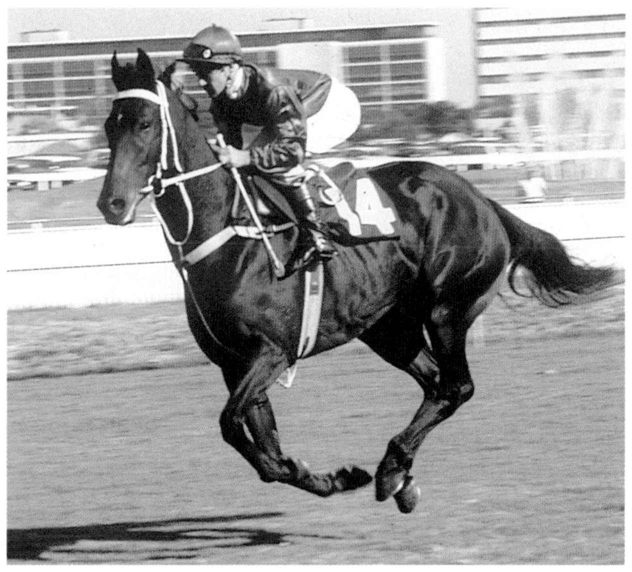

Healthy horses are winners

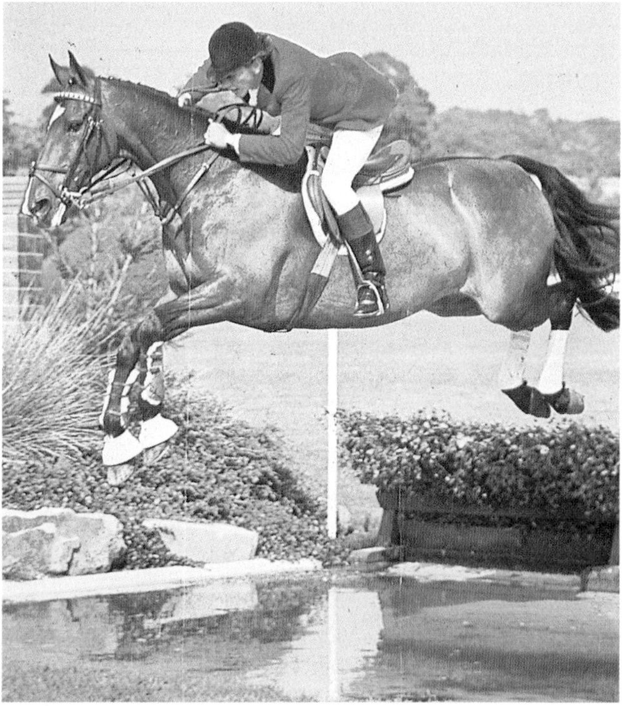

A healthy horse in action

2 metres. Is it rapid or slow, irregular or rhythmical, shallow or deep, light or heavy, noisy or quiet? It will vary according to the horse's fitness, exercise, excitement and temperature of the day. Rapid, irregular, noisy, shallow or heavy respiration is abnormal and requires veterinary attention. Breathing rate can be detected by gently placing the hand over one nostril and feeling the air movement, or by observation of rib or nostril movement.

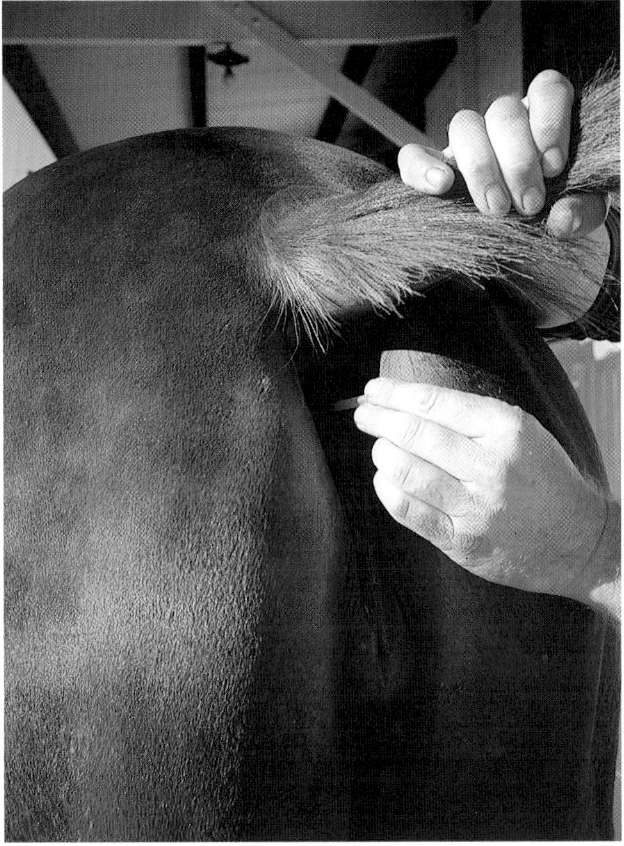

Taking the temperature

## Temperature

A normal thermometer lubricated with vaseline can be used to take the horse's temperature. Insert it through the anus into the rectum for about two-thirds of its length, making sure the bowl of the thermometer is resting against the rectal wall by holding the end of the thermometer to one side after insertion. Leave the thermometer in place for about 1 minute. A horse's normal temperature should range from 37.7°C to 38.6°C. To read the thermometer, hold it between thumb and index finger, rolling it slowly backwards and forwards to enable you to see where the mercury column ends.

You can get a false reading if the mercury is not shaken down before inserting the thermometer or if the thermometer bowl is inserted into a faecal mass rather than being positioned to rest against the rectal wall.

## Urine

Normal urine can vary markedly to the eye; it can be clear and colourless, cloudy and yellow, like water or thick syrup in consistency. Abnormal signs that usually indicate a problem are constant dribbling, no urine passed for 24 hours, an excessive amount passed, urine reddish-brown or blood-tinged in colour. If you suspect something is wrong, collect a sample of urine in a clean jar and place it in the refrigerator for the veterinarian to examine when he arrives.

# WHEN TO CALL YOUR VETERINARIAN

## CALL IMMEDIATELY

**Choke**

Distressed – extends head and neck – salivates – coughs – grunts – paws ground – food and saliva may be regurgitated through nostrils.

**Collapse or loss of balance**

Over-reaction to external stimuli – depression – staggering – knuckling over – walking in circles – down, unable to get up – general muscle tremor – rigidity – paddling movements of legs – coma.

**Continual straining**

Attempting to defaecate (pass a motion) or urinate with little or no result.

**Heavy bleeding**

From any part of body – will not stop – apply pressure.

**Difficulty in breathing**

Gasping – noisy breathing.

**Inability to foal**

If no foal appears after about 25 minutes of obvious contractions and straining – if mare gives up after straining for 20 minutes – if part of foal appears, e.g. leg, but nothing else appears after 20 minutes of straining.

**Injury**

Severe continuous pain – severe lameness – cut with bone exposed – puncture wound especially chest or abdomen.

**Pain**

Severe, continuous or spasmodic.

**Poisoning**

Chemical, snake or plant – retain for veterinarian to identify quickly type of poisoning.

**Urine or diarrhoea**

Evidence of blood – putrid, fluid diarrhoea in young foal.

## CALL SAME DAY

**Abortion**

**Afterbirth**
If retained for 8 hours.

**Breathing difficulties**
Laboured breathing (heaving) – rapid and shallow breathing with or without cough.

**Diarrhoea**
Motion fluid, putrid.

**Eye problem**
Tears streaming down cheeks – eyelids partially or completely closed – cornea (surface of eye) hazy, opaque or bluish-white in colour.

**Injuries**
Not urgent but liable to become infected – a cut through full thickness of skin which needs stitching – puncture wound of foot – sudden acute lameness.

**Itching**
Self-mutilating – damaged skin – bleeding sores.

**Not eating**
Depressed – in conjunction with other signs such as – laboured breathing, diarrhoea, lying down, pain, sweating.

**Swelling**
Hot, hard and painful or discharging.

## CALL WITHIN TWENTY-FOUR HOURS

**Diarrhoea**
Cow-like – no indication of abdominal pain – no sign of blood – no straining.

**Itching**
Moderate – no damage by self-mutilation.

**Lameness**
Ability to bear weight on leg – not affecting eating or other functions.

**Not eating**
No other sign or symptom.

# FIRST AID

The horse's ability to react suddenly and run quickly was its greatest means of protection from predators or danger in earlier days. Even now, when a horse senses danger or is frightened, it will often react in a wild, violent, blind panic, having no regard for ropes, fences or any other objects in its path. Consequently, it often suffers a variety of self-inflicted wounds and damages its body. While exercising, especially at gallop, a horse can cause great damage to itself, particularly to its limbs. The horse is also subject to hurt through incorrect handling, stabling and shoeing.

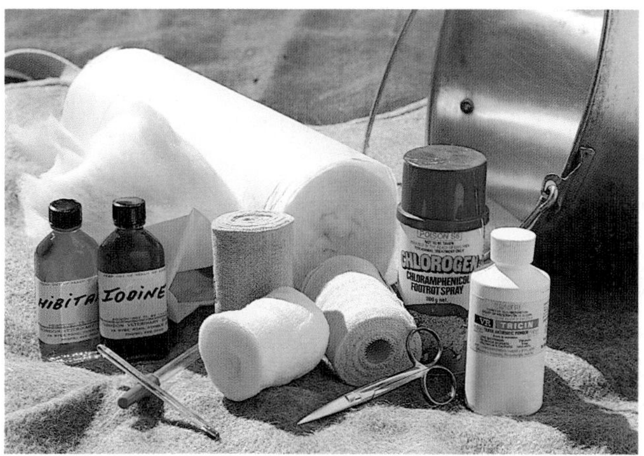

First aid kit

## First aid kit

- Scissors
- Roll of gauze bandage (50 mm)
- Roll of Elastoplast (75 mm)
- Roll of cotton-wool
- Antiseptic wash (e.g. Hibitane)
- Crepe cotton bandages (75 mm)
- Antibiotic powder
- Antibiotic pressure pak spray
- Clean bucket
- Thermometer
- Tincture of iodine

## First aid for bleeding, wounds, fractures, collapse (shock)

### *Bleeding*

First step in treating any wound is to control haemorrhage (bleeding) – if blood slowly oozing from wound, apply direct pressure to site by means of piece of clean gauze or sheeting held between fingers – don't dab or wipe wound – tends to promote further bleeding – hold pressure on wound for 10 seconds – remove hand holding gauze or sheeting – evaluate depth and breadth of wound – if bleeding recommences, apply further pressure.

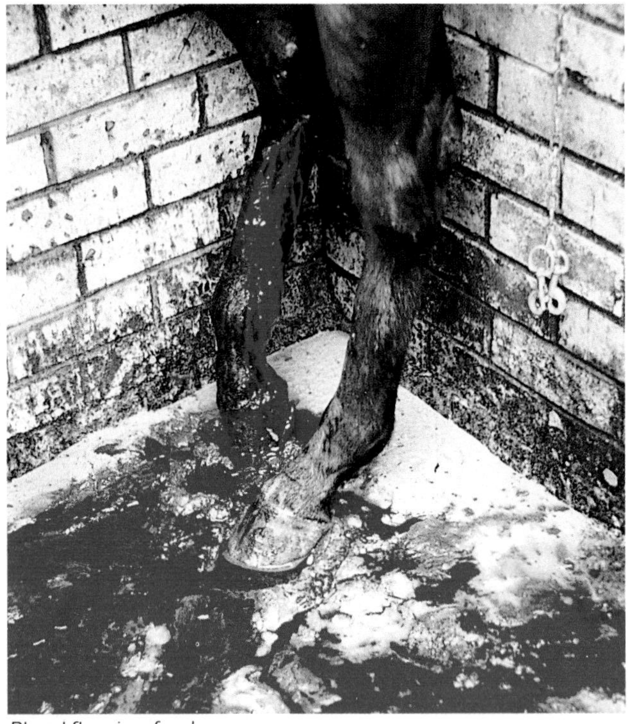

Blood flowing freely

If blood not oozing but flowing freely – take wad of gauze or suitable absorbent material and apply heavy pressure to wound with clean hand – over wad of gauze, wrap firmly but not too tightly 75 mm wide Elastoplast – leave it in place for about 30 minutes – remove bandage and evaluate wound – do not use cotton-wool because small, fine fibres tend to collect in wound, act as foreign body and slow down healing process.

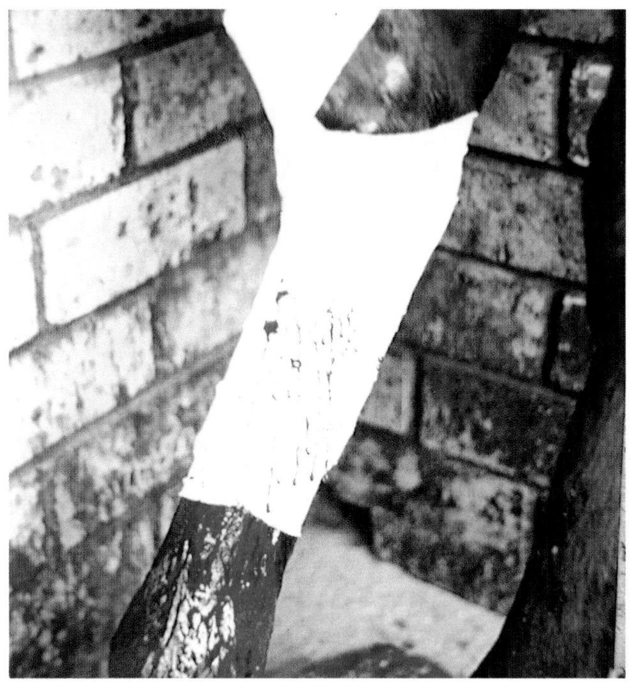

A firmly applied Elastoplast bandage controls the haemorrhage

In cases of arterial bleeding, blood is normally bright red and spurts out with pulsating action – apply very heavy pressure with gauze in hand directly over site of bleeding – wrap 75 mm wide Elastoplast tightly around gauze – not only does bandage apply pressure, but it also immobilises edges of wound, thereby helping to stop bleeding – movement of horse stimulates blood flow and indirectly quickens bleeding – if horse is bleeding, keep it calm and quiet, preferably tied up in a stall – leave bandage in place and call your veterinarian for further advice.

When horse is bleeding from inaccessible area such as inside nostrils, restrict its movement – externally apply cold to area in form of slowly running water from hose or ice packed in a towel.

To sum up – don't stand and watch a horse bleed to death – immediately apply direct pressure and stop horse from moving about.

Tourniquets are not recommended – often difficult to apply – if applied incorrectly can accentuate rather than retard blood loss.

## *Wounds*

Most wounds seen in horses are contaminated – because of horse's susceptibility to infection, your veterinary surgeon should be consulted about tetanus injection and treatment with antibiotics. There are several types of wounds:

ABRASIONS

Normally painful to touch – haemorrhage a little – often contaminated with grit and dirt – can be removed by directing running water from hose with firm pressure onto wound – careful about pressure – if too severe may tend to drive foreign material further into tissues.

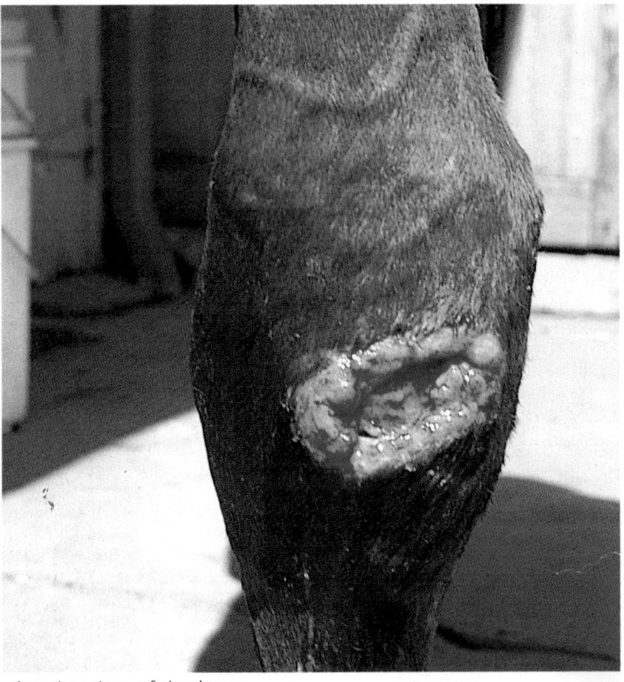

An abrasion of the knee

As an alternative, wound may be cleaned with peroxide, which has germicidal as well as foaming action that helps flush out debris.

Once wound is clean, pat it dry with clean gauze and dust it with antibiotic powder, paint it with gentian violet or spray it with one of the aerosol packs containing antibiotics and triple dye – leave abrasion open unless oozing freely, in which case cover with gauze bandage – if abrasion covers large area, do not exercise horse until healing is obvious.

CONTUSIONS

These wounds are characterised by bruising and swelling of skin and underlying tissues – not necessarily associated with break in skin – a break is an excellent environment for development of bacteria – antibiotics are essential, no matter how small the break.

If no abrasion or break in skin, swelling best dealt with by application of alternate hot and cold foments – to make a hot foment, put hot water into bucket containing 2 tablespoons of salt – water should be just hot enough for your hand to tolerate it – remember: if water is too hot, it will scald horse's skin – if too cold, will not serve purpose of increasing blood circulation to the area – blood aids in repair of damaged tissue and carries away debris and damaged cells.

Drop large wad of cotton-wool into bucket containing hot water – hold it on contused area until it cools off – repeat procedure for 10 minutes, morning and night – be sure that water is kept at same temperature during 10-minute procedure.

To apply cold foment, hose wounded area with fair amount of water pressure – cold water constricts blood vessels, reduces oozing of fluid into contused area – pressure has a massaging effect, stimulating circulation and flow of fluid away from the site.

PUNCTURE WOUNDS

Puncture wounds may or may not be accompanied by haemorrhage – generally painful – to treat, clean site of puncture thoroughly with an iodine based scrub or

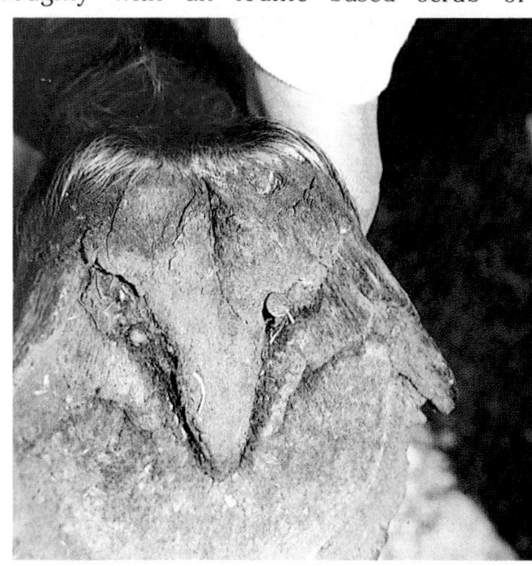

Nail puncture

Hibiclens – remove any dirt, debris or dead tissue – try to make opening to puncture as large as possible to allow proper drainage – always check wound carefully to see that no foreign body remains embedded – any remnant of foreign body left in the wound will delay healing process – finally, paint opening and as far into puncture as possible with tincture of iodine – after wound has been cleansed and sterilised, it should be kept open as long as possible while drainage is taking place – horse should be given hot foments to relieve pain and aid healing.

Administration of antibiotics and anti-tetanus vaccine are necessary precautions in treatment of puncture wounds – many puncture wounds go unnoticed – if infection or dirty foreign bodies are lying in or underneath skin, an abscess will probably form – contact your veterinary surgeon who will provide necessary drainage, antibiotics and anti-tetanus vaccine.

### LACERATIONS

Lacerations are not usually acutely painful and haemorrhage is variable according to type of blood vessels that have been severed.

Treatment can be complicated – clean wound thoroughly by hosing or application of peroxide – remove any hair, dead tissue or foreign bodies – apply antibiotic powder, zinc cream, or a mild astringent to exposed flesh – beware of strong antiseptics that not only fail to destroy bacteria but will irritate wound, destroying important cells necessary for wound healing.

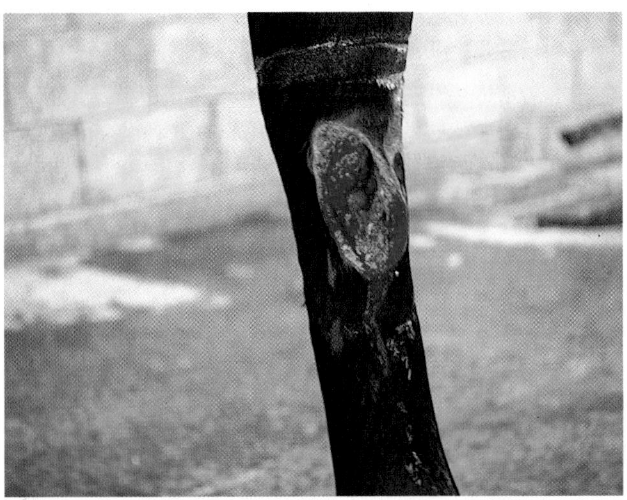

A laceration

If one of horse's legs has been lacerated, cover wound with gauze held in position by a firmly applied Elastoplast bandage – if pressure of bandage too tight, blood supply to area will be impaired, slowing down wound healing. A firm pressure bandage controls swelling – helps to immobilise wound edges – stops production of proud flesh – if leg does not swell, leave bandage on for 2 days.

When bandage is removed, it will be soggy and discoloured with discharge from wound – odour probably offensive – this is normal, provided horse is on a good antibiotic cover – hose wound – clean away any discharge, debris or dead tissue – dress as before – continue process just described until fleshy tissue has filled in the cavity to skin level – leave off bandages, allowing air and sunshine to dry surface of wound.

Do not exercise the horse – confine to stable or yard until skin has completely covered wound.

### INCISED WOUNDS

Characteristics of these wounds are – edges are clean cut, fairly well-opposed – minimum tissue damage.

If you think wound needs stitching you should call your veterinarian straight away – for good healing it should be stitched within 8 hours of accident.

## *Fractures*

If a horse has obvious fracture of lower limb, apply a splint to prevent any further damage at site of fracture while waiting for veterinarian – splint can be readily made by wrapping pillow or roll of cotton-wool around leg, with fracture in the centre of cotton-wool or pillow – bind pillow or cotton-wool to leg with crepe bandages applied as tightly as possible – to add extra rigidity, a broom handle is incorporated in bandage, with a final few layers of 75 mm Elastoplast applied as tightly as possible – splint not only immobilises fracture – also helps relieve certain amount of pain.

## *Collapse (shock)*

Shock is term used to describe state of collapse – follows many forms of serious stress such as car accidents, massive haemorrhage, heavy falls, overwhelming infection (septicaemia), twisted bowel (colic) and dehydration – symptoms can vary – depending on cause, include depression, prostration, rapid breathing and pallor of gums and conjunctiva (membranes around eye).

Contact veterinarian immediately – while waiting for his

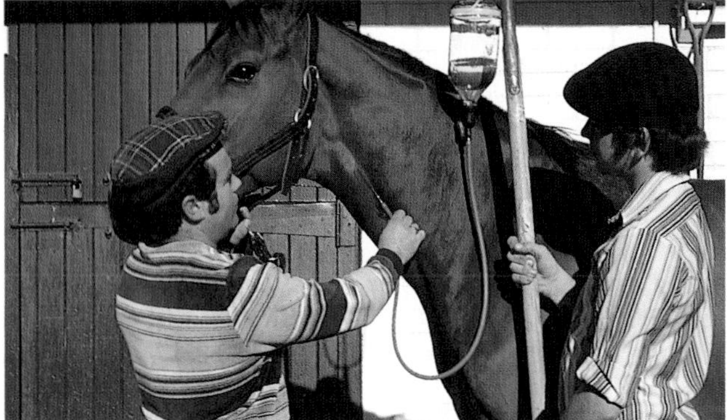
A shocked horse receives a transfusion of fluids and electrolytes

arrival, take following steps:

- Keep horse warm but not too warm, i.e. maintain normal body temperature – warmth can be overdone to point of accentuating shock if horse becomes too hot.
- Control any bleeding (see page 32).
- Ask people nearby to be quiet or move away – noisy group of spectators can aggravate shock.
- Keep horse calm and quiet by tying it up or putting it in a stall – if it is lying outstretched, spasmodically struggling to get up but unable to do so, rather than letting it flounder with risk of further injury, put a head collar and lead on it and prevent it from getting up by kneeling on extended neck and head with your full weight.

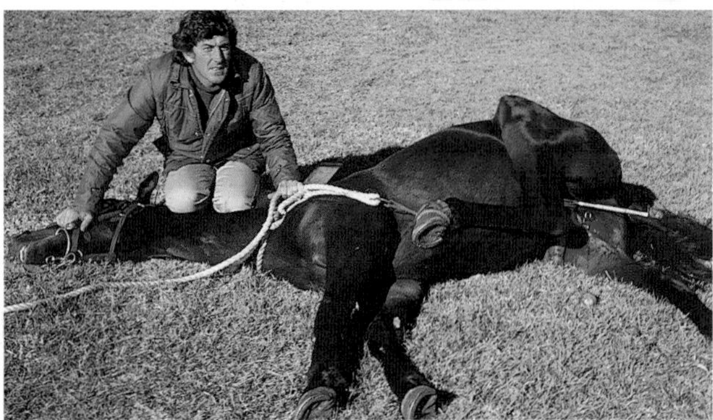
A horse is prevented from standing if its extended neck is knelt on

## Bandaging hints

Suitable bandages for first aid are a plaster bandage with an adhesive surface 75 mm wide or a cotton crepe bandage 75 mm wide – before any wound is bandaged cover it with gauze – do not use cotton-wool – small, fine fibres tend to collect in wound, act as foreign body and slow down healing process.

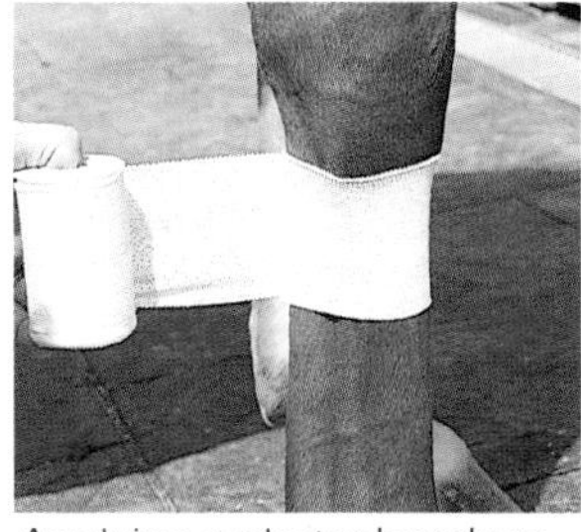

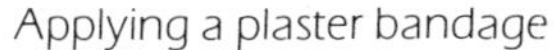

Applying a plaster bandage

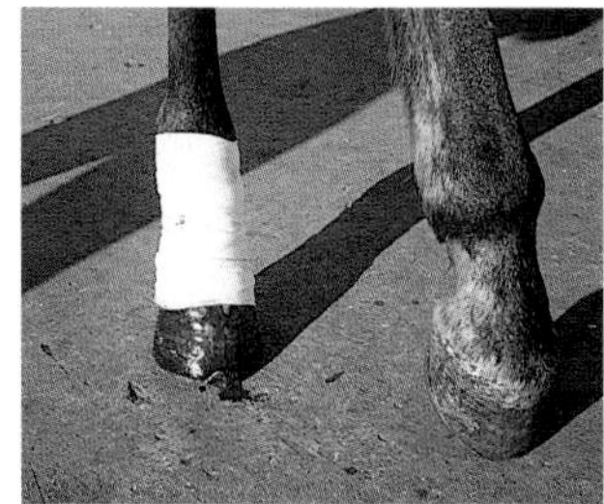

Bandaging completed

Do not fall into trap of applying plaster bandage too tightly – unroll manageable part of bandage then wrap that part round leg, unroll another part, continue likewise. If you unroll as you wrap, bandage will invariably be too tight – as you apply plaster bandage and blood is soaking through or seeping under it wrap more layers of bandage more tightly until blood flow stops (see bleeding, page 32).

When applying cotton crepe bandage leave about 75 mm of bandage as flap – wrap bandage round the leg in clockwise direction, overlapping each round by half – after first time round, draw down flap and secure it by wrapping bandage over it as you continue – when you come to end of bandage, secure it with clips, safety pins or strip of adhesive plaster.

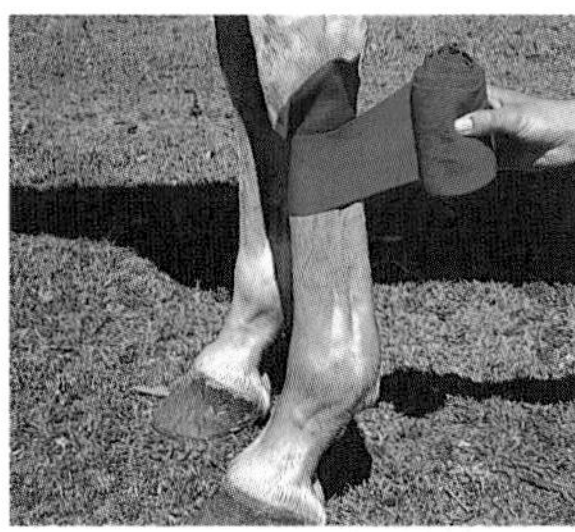

Applying a cotton crepe bandage, leaving about 75 mm as flap

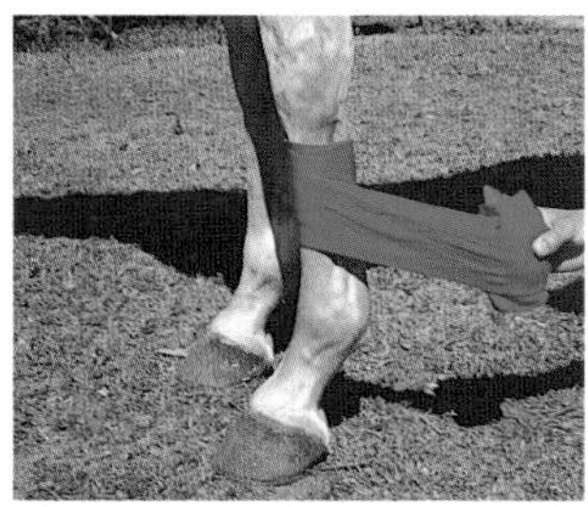

Drawing the flap down and wrapping the bandage over it

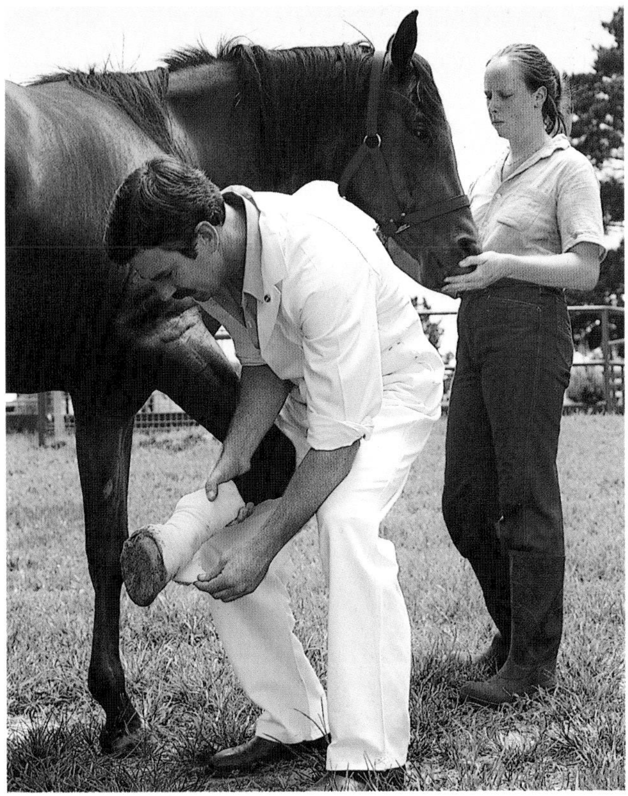

Face the rear of the horse when bandaging

Always stand to the side of the leg, facing hindquarters, to put on or take off bandage – stoop over or bend knees, but never kneel down.

The beginning and end of all bandaging should be secure – bandages that slip and/or unravel don't perform their function and can be dangerous.

Apply bandage with firm, even pressure – check to see that leg does not swell – if it does, it is a sign that bandage has been applied too tightly – remove and re-apply.

Cotton-wool under bandages can sometimes form hard balls that act as pressure points – layers of sponge rubber under bandage will ensure an even distribution of pressure – uneven pressure over a tendon can produce a bow in it.

Before applying a bandage around knee joint – first feel bone under skin at back of knee towards outside – do not cover bone with bandage – otherwise nasty pressure sore may develop.

# ADMINISTERING MEDICATION

There is nothing more frustrating and worrying than refusal of medication by a horse. If medication is not administered correctly, the horse's condition will not improve and may worsen, and in most cases the medicine is wasted. If you find it impossible to medicate your horse, a veterinarian can administer medication in an uncomplicated manner. Whether medicine is given orally, by stomach tube, by injection or via the rectum depends upon type of medicine, palatability, speed of onset and duration of its action, condition and temperament of the horse and temperament of the owner.

## Oral administration of drugs

### *Pelleted preparations in feed*

Numerous vitamin and mineral supplements, worm preparations, etc, are pelleted to prevent wastage and have additives such as flavouring to make them palatable. They can be mixed in as part of the normal feed.

### *Powders and liquids in feed*

Provided these are palatable, they can be thoroughly mixed with feed so that the horse cannot selectively avoid the powder or liquid and eat the remainder of the food. Powders tend to collect in the bottom of the feed bin in inaccessible corners and when the horse is eating it tends to blow its nostrils into the feed, causing some of the powder to be blown out of the feed bin. If powder and liquid preparations are not palatable, they can be mixed with molasses or honey, then mixed with the feed or placed on a large wooden spoon and wiped over the horse's tongue.

### *Powders and liquids in drinking water*

Many electrolyte mixtures in powdered form can be given in drinking water. Leave the horse in the yard or stable for a number of hours without water. Add powder to a bucket about a quarter full of water and offer it to the horse. When it has finished drinking top up the bucket with fresh water.

### *Liquids and pastes by syringe*

Many worming pastes are now packaged in a syringe. Put a head collar on the horse with lead attached, then make sure the mouth is empty before introducing the syringe.

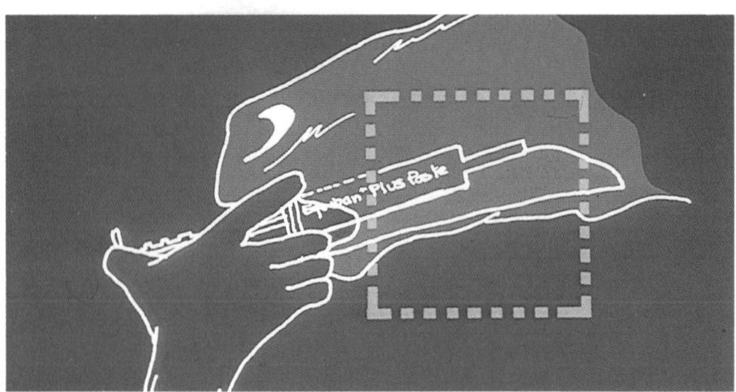

Administering paste in a syringe

Stand on the left side of the horse's head, facing the horse, and put the syringe in the corner of the mouth so that the nozzle rests on the back of the tongue. After pressing plunger of syringe, ensure that the full dose is swallowed by holding up the horse's head, but not too high so that the horse will have no difficulty in swallowing.

If the syringe contains a liquid, don't squirt it rapidly onto the back of the tongue, as some may go into the windpipe and cause inhalation pneumonia. Gently dribble it onto the tongue, allowing sufficient time for the horse to swallow.

## *Tablets, capsules and boluses placed in the mouth*

These can be given by hand or with a balling gun. A gag may be used, but it is not necessary. If one is used, it can be applied in the same way as a bridle. It has the advantage of opening the mouth wide so that the tablet can be placed in the very back of the mouth without finger, hand or arm being bitten or abraded.

To administer medication by hand without a gag, stand on the left (near side) of the horse's head, facing the horse.

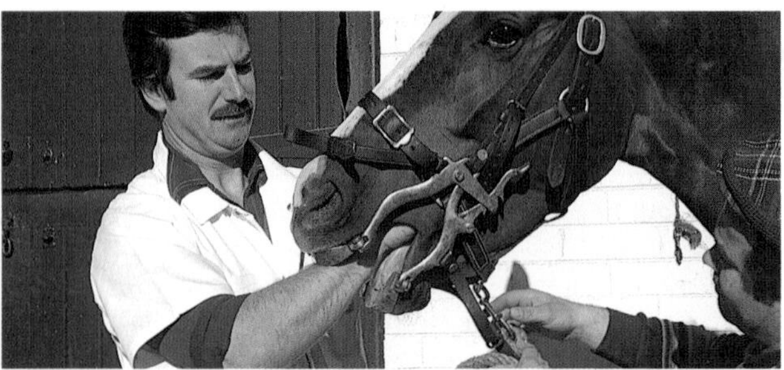

Using a gag to administer medication by hand

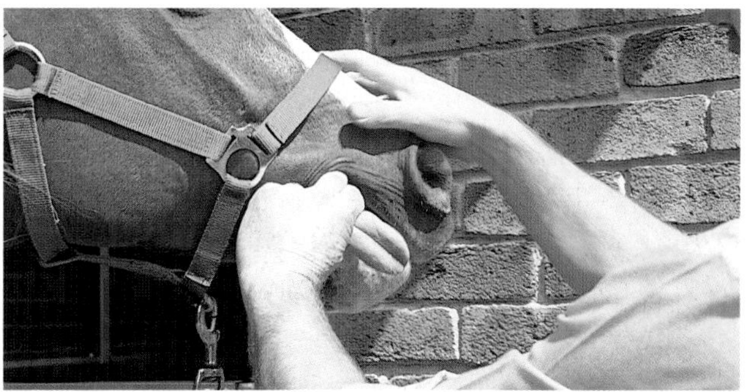

Grasping the tongue before administering medication

Putting your left hand into the right side of the horse's mouth, grasp a good handful of the tongue and pull it out between the lips on the right side of mouth. As well as keeping the mouth open, this will stop the horse from biting your hand because it will bite its own tongue first. With your right hand, place tablet, capsule or bolus as far back on tongue as possible and quickly release the tongue that you are holding. This action carries the tablet into the back of the throat. Lubricating the tablet before introducing it and holding the horse's head in a slightly elevated position helps the tablet to slide down more smoothly.

Using the balling gun to administer medication, grasp the tongue as described above, introduce the gun between the incisor (front) teeth, discharging bolus or capsule onto the base of the tongue. If it is discharged too far to the back of the mouth, damage can be done to the throat. Do not put irritant materials in gelatine capsules as sometimes they become caught in throat or oesophagus (food pipe), dissolve and release irritant material with risk of causing severe local damage.

## *Drenching with bottle in mouth*

To carry out this procedure, elevate the horse's head sufficiently to allow the liquid to flow to the back of the throat. If the head cannot be held high enough by hand, attach a rope to the noseband of the head collar and raise the head by pulling on a rope thrown over a rafter. A plastic bottle with a long neck is introduced into the mouth where there is a gap between the teeth. Slowly trickle the solution into the horse's mouth, allowing plenty of time to swallow. There is the danger of fluid getting into the windpipe, causing secondary pneumonia, so remember to drench slowly with a bottle.

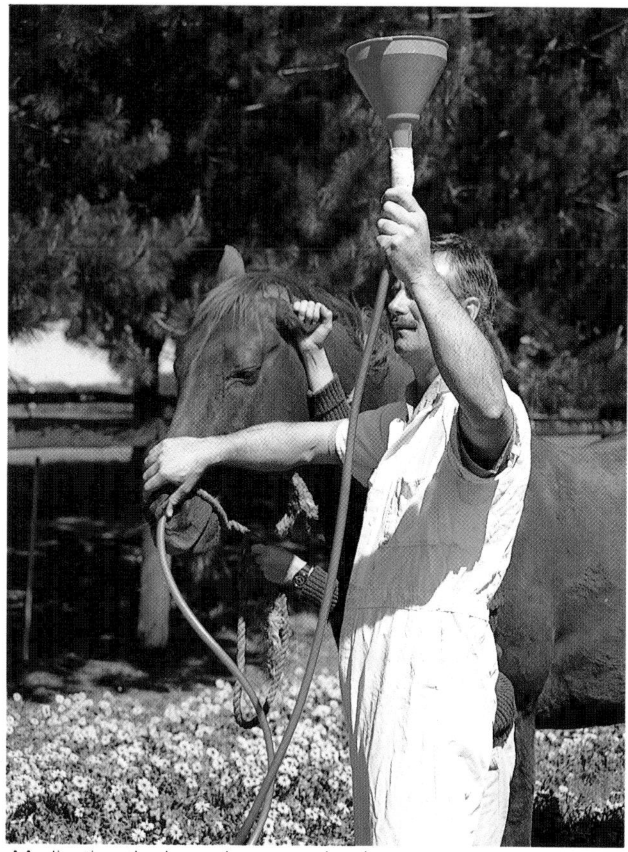
Medicating the horse by stomach tube

## Nasal administration of drugs

The stomach tube is an efficient, safe, professional method of giving liquid medication, but I feel use of this technique should be left to the veterinary surgeon or trained personnel. In inexperienced hands, many horses have died from the stomach tube inadvertently being passed into the lungs, resulting in fatal inhalation pneumonia.

## Administration of drugs by injection

This procedure is often used by veterinary surgeons as it is quick, efficient and convenient. Injections can be given under the skin (subcutaneous), into muscle (intramuscular), into a vein (intravenous) or into a joint space (intra-articular). The type of drug used and the disease being treated determine how and where the injection will

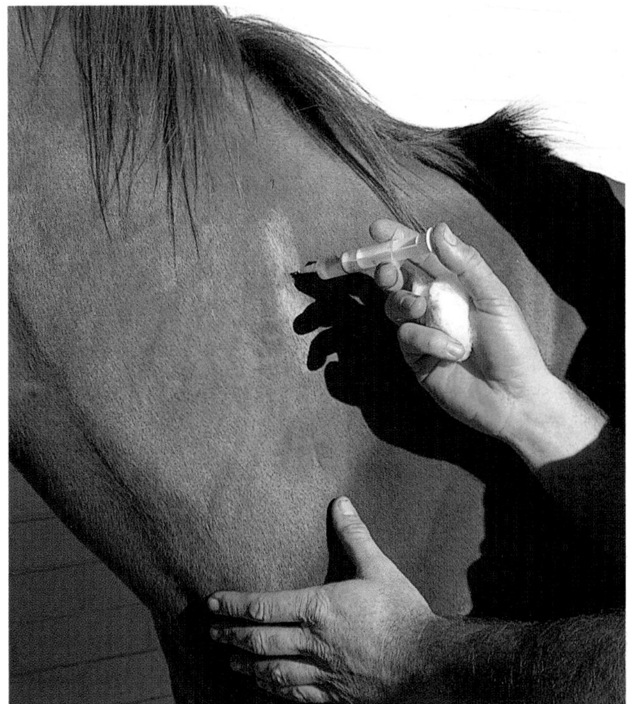

Intramuscular injection

be given. This technique should be employed only by veterinary surgeons or trained personnel.

## Administration of drugs via rectum

Extreme care should be taken when giving an enema to a foal. Use a soft tube and make sure it is well lubricated. Do not insert tube more than 10 cm into rectum, and insert it gently. Allow the fluid to flow by gravity; this is much safer than forcing it in under pressure because of the risk of rupturing the rectal wall.

## Administering bran mash

Sick horses are prone to constipation. Bran mash can be used to encourage a sick or convalescent horse to eat, as well as being an effective means of treating and preventing constipation.

To make bran mash: place 1 kg of bran, 30 grams of salt and 300 ml of molasses into a clean bucket; add 2 litres of hot water and stir thoroughly. Allow mixture to stand for 10 minutes before offering it to the horse.

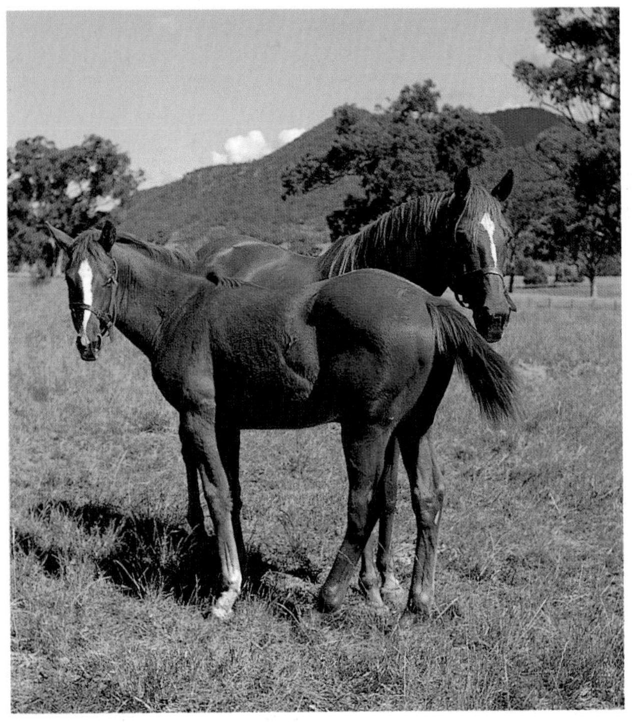

Healthy mare and foal

# SIGNS OF DISEASES AND HEALTH PROBLEMS A–Z

1. Look in the index at the beginning of this section to find the first sign of the disease or health problem that you have observed in your horse. Turn to the page reference given.

2. Read the groups of associated signs that are listed under the first sign observed by you and select the group that applies most closely to your horse. It will give you the possible diagnosis of your horse's problem and a page reference. Turn to it.

3. Keep in mind that all the signs associated with a disease or health problem may not be observed all at once. Some may not be seen at any stage; others may be observed in sequence as the complaint develops.

# INDEX OF SIGNS OF DISEASES

# ABDOMINAL PAIN

Find below the group of associated signs that best fits what you observe in your horse.

## ASSOCIATED SIGNS

► Foal cannot pass motion – signs of straining – appears constipated – becomes colicky – no anal opening.

Possible diagnosis: Atresia Ani – *see page 159*

---

► Pain less severe and more continuous than in spasmodic colic – abdomen enlarges noticeably in upper right flank – small amount of dung and gas passed.

Possible diagnosis: Colic: flatulent – *see page 177*

---

► History of eating large quantities of wheat, maize, coarse straw, young clover, mouldy grain or hay – greedy overfeeding. Severe abdominal pain – swollen abdomen when tapped with fingers has a drum-like sound and feel – horse kicks at abdomen – throws itself on ground – rapid panting-type breathing – sweats profusely – mucous membranes around eyes and gums vary from brick red to bluish colour – breath is sour – horse may adopt dog-sitting position – vomiting rare. If stomach ruptures – horse quietens down – its temperature falls – goes into shock – can die suddenly.

Possible diagnosis: Colic: gastric dilatation – *see page 177*

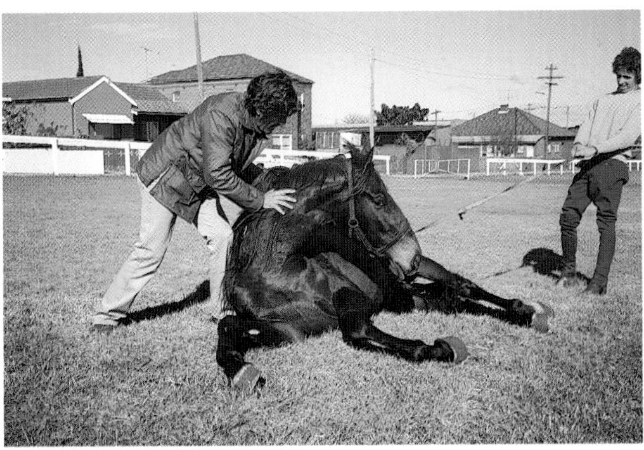

Trying to get a horse with abdominal pain to its feet

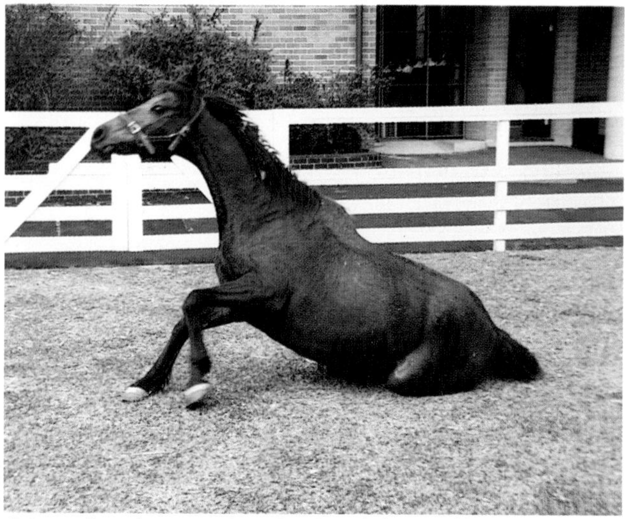

A horse in pain may adopt the dog-sitting position

► Develops slowly – abdominal pain may disappear for day or two then reappear more violently – dung passed in small quantities, drier, harder than usual.

Possible diagnosis: Colic: impaction – *see page 178*

---

► In early stages, violent pain associated with increased intestinal sounds – hours later no intestinal sounds heard. Rapid respiration and heart rate – sweating – dehydration – mucous membrane of gum and eye brick red to bluish to white – shock sets in.

Possible diagnosis: Colic: obstruction – *see page 179*

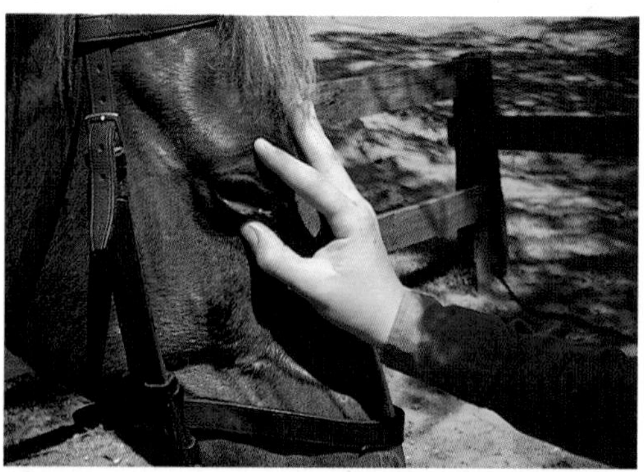

The mucous membrane of the eye is brick red

► Spasm of intestine gives rise to severe abdominal pain – indicated by such signs as stamping hind feet – kicking at belly – in extreme cases, horse becomes violent – intervals of calm between signs – calm periods less frequent as pain lengthens and intensifies. Frequent, rapid, loud intestinal sounds can be heard.

Possible diagnosis: Colic: spasmodic – *see page 180*

---

► Foal strains without results – often observed 12–18 hours after birth – throws itself to ground and thrashes violently.

Possible diagnosis: Constipation – *see page 183*

---

► Sudden onset of abdominal pain – often after exhausting exercise – repeated straining to urinate – little or no urine passed – possible presence of blood and/or sand-like deposits in urine – skin around vulva and between legs of mares may be scalded due to dribbling urine.

Possible diagnosis: Cystitis, Kidney Stones or Bladder Stones – page 191

---

► *Horse:* Dung cow-like, or like porridge or discoloured water – signs of discomfort when passing motion – swishing tail – looking at flank – tucking up abdomen. *Foal:* Dung fluid and putrid – straining – tucking up abdomen. Can cause death.

Possible diagnosis: Diarrhoea – *see page 195–6*

---

► Mare's abdomen large and swollen – sweating – restless – agitated – pawing ground – stretching – swishing

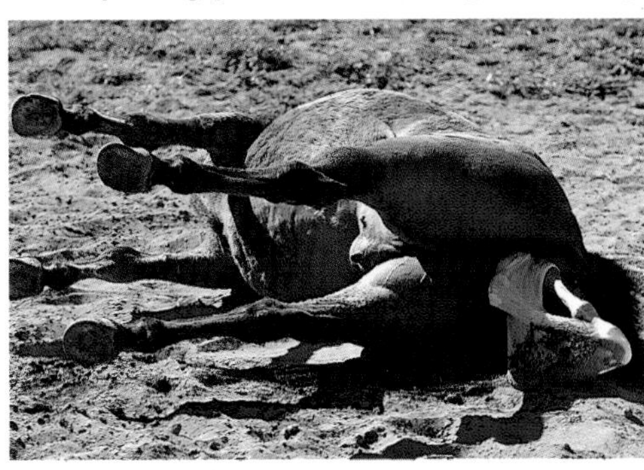

Foaling

tail – lying down – getting up – fluid from vagina – straining – foetal membrane appears at vagina.

Possible diagnosis: Foaling (parturition) – *see page 205*

---

► Temperature rise – disinclined to move – wants to be down but reluctant – grunting associated with breathing – abdominal muscles tense – loss of appetite and weight – dehydration.

Possible diagnosis: Peritonitis – *see page 260*

---

► Abdominal pain – diarrhoea – wobbly gait (staggering) – depression – twitching – grinding teeth – slobbering from mouth – paralysis – convulsions – collapse – access to poisons or poisonous plants.

Possible diagnosis: Poisoning – *see page 262*

---

► Foal shows signs of depression 12–24 hours after birth – strains repeatedly to urinate – very little or no urine passed – straining can be similar in constipated foal – do not confuse.

Possible diagnosis: Ruptured Bladder – *see page 273*

# ABORTION

Find below the group of associated signs that best fits what you observe in your horse.

## BACKGROUND

Abortion is defined as the abnormal expulsion of the foetus, dead or alive, from first month to full term of pregnancy. Abortion in the first 30 days of pregnancy cannot be substantiated because accurate diagnosis of pregnancy is difficult. If embryo dies it is generally reabsorbed by the mare; if expelled it is possibly not noticed because of its small size and gelatinous nature.

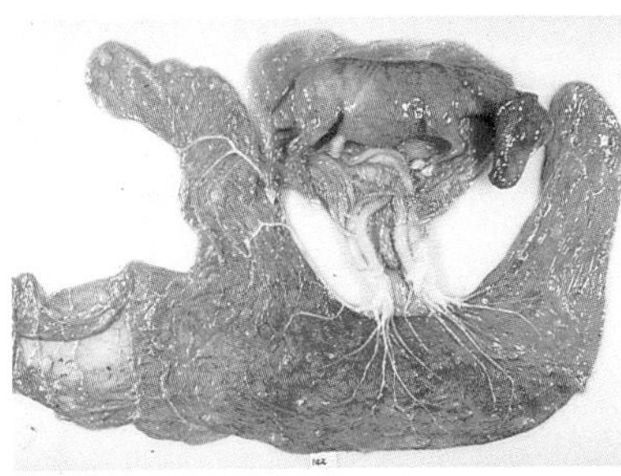

This foetus was aborted about 26 weeks after conception

If mare aborts, transfer other mares to another paddock. Do not move mare, foetus or foetal membrane till veterinarian takes tissue samples and swabs mare, then burn or bury remains. Isolate mare till veterinarian test results are known. Disinfect with Hibitane or similar preparation the area where the abortion took place. Staff handling the mare or aborted foetus should wash hands thoroughly, disinfect boots and change clothes before handling other horses, especially pregnant mares.

## ASSOCIATED SIGNS

- Usually occurs before 150th day of pregnancy but possible at any stage – premature foal unable to suck – weak and dull. Often retention of placenta and vaginal discharge – history of contact with cattle (brucellosis) and pigs (leptospirosis).

Possible diagnosis: Abortion: bacterial – *see page 151*

---

- Occurs about 10th month of pregnancy – swab and culture by veterinarian show signs of fungi.

Possible diagnosis: Abortion: fungal infection – *see page 151*

► May occur between 3rd and 5th month – low levels of hormone, progesterone, known to cause abortion at certain stages of pregnancy – mare may have history of abortions unrelated to infection or other causes.

Possible diagnosis: Abortion: hormonal – *see page 152*

---

► Severe stress – excitement – trauma – prolonged lack of feed and drinking water – distant and tiring transport especially during 90–160th day of pregnancy – excessive exercise.

Possible diagnosis: Abortion: stress – *see page 152*

---

► Abortion of two foetuses – most common between 5th and 9th months.

Possible diagnosis: Abortion: twinning – *see page 152*

---

► (a) Incubation period of infection about 2 weeks – symptoms of a cold – temperature up – nasal discharge – coughing – sneezing – respiratory disease – abortion may occur up to 4 months after infection when mare appears healthy – abortion usually occurs from 5th month onwards. Foetus expelled rapidly with placenta – virus can affect brain and spinal cord of mare causing paralysis of hindquarters – foetus aborted after 6 months shows discolouration of placental fluid and hooves due to diarrhoea in uterus. Disease found throughout world including Australia.

Possible diagnosis: Abortion: viral (Equine Herpes Virus I; Equine Viral Rhinopneumonitis) – *see page 153*

---

► (b) Pregnant mares may abort during illness or shortly after – incubation period of 2–6 days – symptoms may be high temperature (42°C) – off food – dopey – weak – inflamed, discoloured eyes – nasal discharge. Some show oedema (swelling) in legs, udder and underbelly – constipation – colic – diarrhoea.

Possible diagnosis: Abortion: viral (Equine Viral Arteritis) – *see page 153*

# BREATHING NOISE

Find below the group of associated signs that best fits what you observe in your horse.

## ASSOCIATED SIGNS

► A peculiar noise, ranging from a whistle to a roar, that some horses make when they breathe in (inspiration) – most horses only show signs of the noise when galloping fully extended – a minority show signs even at rest. Horse's ability to perform in events where there is stress on respiratory system is adversely affected – occurs most often in horses 16 hands or more in height and aged 3–7 years – rare in ponies.

Possible diagnosis: Roaring (Laryngeal Hemiplegia) – *see page 272*

---

► Noise during strenuous exercise, e.g. extended gallop – often towards end of race – horse makes a choking noise – may be associated with breathing in and out.

Possible diagnosis: Soft Palate Displacement – *see page 280*

# BREEDING PROBLEMS (MARE)

Find below the group of associated signs that best fits what you observe in your horse.

## BACKGROUND

About 25% of thoroughbred brood mares do not become pregnant in any one stud season. The causes are numerous, complex and sometimes impossible to identify with certainty. Common causes are infection, structural defects of the vulva, hormonal imbalance, and nutritional and psychological problems.

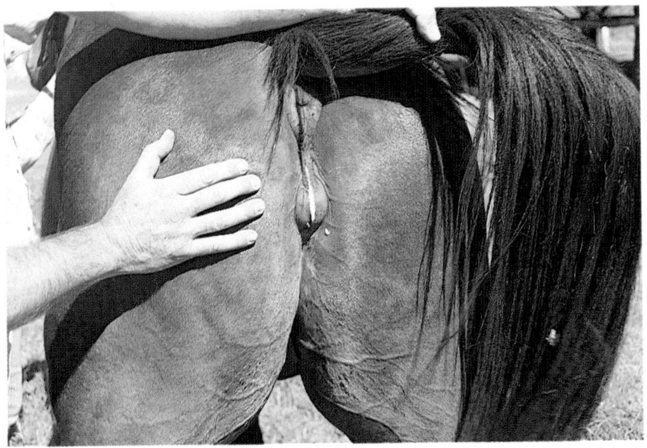

Discharge of pus from vagina — a sign of infection

## ASSOCIATED SIGNS

- During normal breeding season mare may not come into season regularly or fails to show signs of heat – is on heat or in season continuously – has irregular lengths of heat cycles.

Possible diagnosis: Hormonal Imbalance – *see page 224*

---

- Vaginal discharge – failure to conceive or maintain pregnancy – reproductive cycle normal.

Possible diagnosis: Infected Uterus or Contagious Equine Metritis (CEM) – *see page 226 (Infected Uterus) or page 183 (CEM)*

---

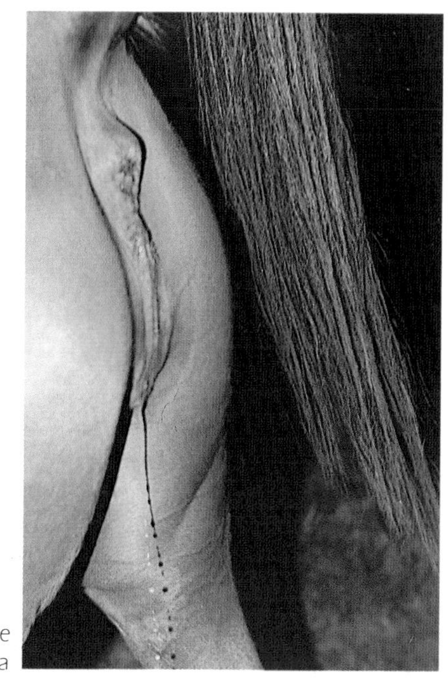
Pus discharge from the vulva

► Symptoms arise 12–24 hours after foaling – temperature rise – lethargy – off food – bloody brown or creamy yellow discharge from vulva – constant drip of blood – laminitis (see page 211) may be evident.

Possible diagnosis: Post-Foaling Metritis – *see page 263*

---

► During normal breeding season shows no signs of heat (oestrus).

Possible diagnosis: Psychological Problems – *see page 264*

---

► Tear through vaginal wall into rectum – occurs in foaling – observed without hindrance if mare's tail lifted out of way to expose anus and vulva.

Possible diagnosis: Recto-Vaginal Fistula – *see page 269*

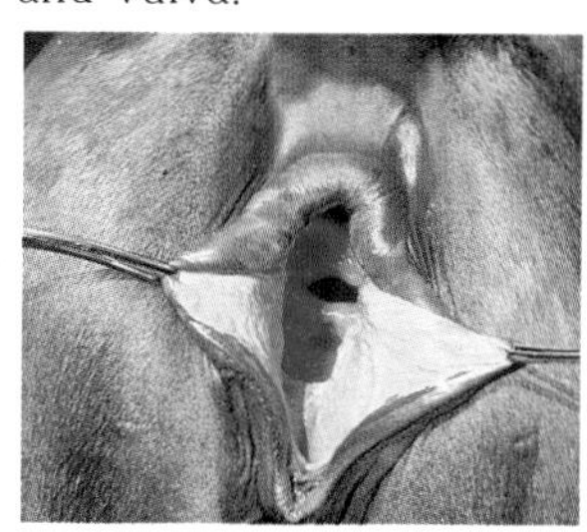
Recto-vaginal fistula caused by the foal's feet during birth

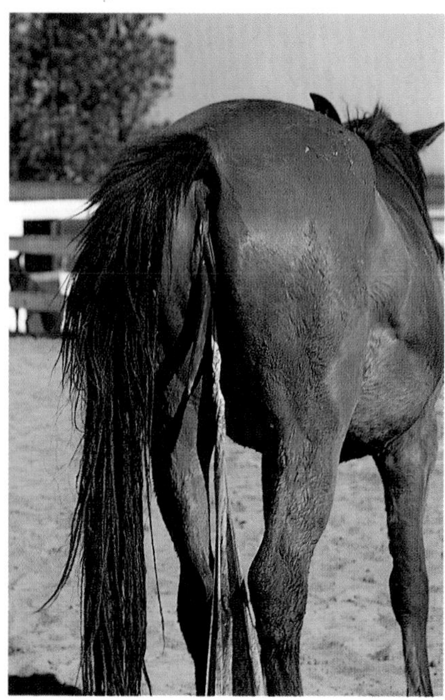

The afterbirth hanging from the mare's vulva

► Foetal membranes (afterbirth) hanging from mare's vulva for more than 8 hours.

Possible diagnosis: Retained afterbirth – *see page 155*

# BREEDING PROBLEMS (STALLION)

Find below the group of associated signs that best fits what you observe in your horse.

## BACKGROUND

There is no more costly and bitter disappointment than finding that your stallion, which you chose so carefully, is infertile. Stallion infertility is a complex problem. It may mean that the horse is unable to produce sperm; or the horse may produce sperm which, for one reason or another, renders the mare it serves infertile (e.g. the stallion is a carrier of contagious equine metritis (CEM).

## ASSOCIATED SIGNS

► Small blister first on head of penis then on its body – blisters develop into pustules – then into ulcers in few days.

Possible diagnosis: Coital Exanthema – *see page 177*

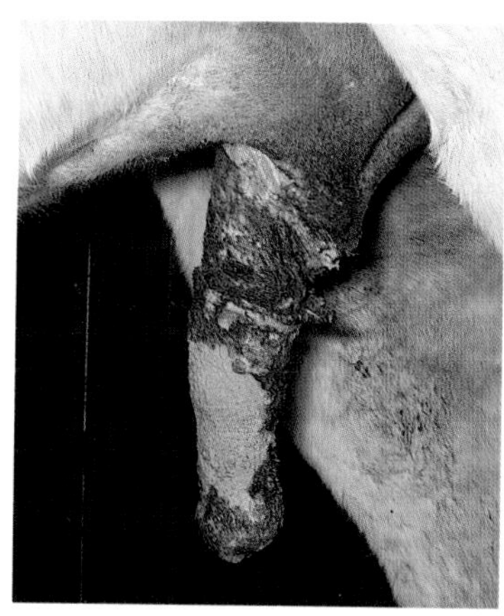

Infected penis

---

► Stallion shows no visible signs of infection – mare after returning to stallion for 2–3 services still not pregnant – mare shows positive swab to CEM.

Possible diagnosis: Contagious Equine Metritis (carrier) – *see page 184*

---

► Encountered mainly in tropics and sub-tropics.

Early stage: swelling of penis and prepuce – genitalia covered with blisters, pustules and ulcers – scrotum and testicles become swollen.

Later stage: weakness of hindquarters – knuckling – stumbling – circular swellings of skin on croup, shoulder, chest and abdomen – 2–4 cm in size – appear and disappear rapidly.

Terminal cases: hypersensitive to touch – ticklishness and paralysis of hindquarters – severe weight loss – stallion lies down.

Possible diagnosis: Dourine – *see page 196*

---

► Small testicles – hard on palpation – poor quality semen – lack of libido. Testes may have failed to descend (cryptorchid) – or only one testicle has descended (monorchid) – such a horse is known as a 'rig'.

Possible diagnosis: Genetic Problems – *see page 215*

---

► Lack of libido (sexual drive).

Possible diagnosis: Hormonal Problems – *see page 224*

---

► Fat, overfed stallion – lacks libido – poor sperm quality – sexually lazy – signs of laminitis (founder, see page 211).

Possible diagnosis: Nutritional Problems – *see page 242*

---

► Acute stage: swelling of scrotum – stiff gait – one or both testicles may be involved – hot and painful if palpated – may refuse to serve mare (breed) – may have temperature rise.

Chronic stage: testes may be of normal size – insensitive to touch – feel harder than normal.

Possible diagnosis: Orchitis – *see page 243*

---

► Masturbation – lack of libido – poor quality semen. Rejection of mare in season for no obvious reason – (may be because of her colour, size, age, odour or some other factor) – 5 minutes later accepts and serves another mare vigorously.

Possible diagnosis: Psychological Problems – *see page 265*

# BURNS

## ASSOCIATED SIGNS

► Blackened hair – swelling of skin and underlying tissues – blisters on skin – dead skin followed by sloughing of skin leaving large denuded areas which ooze a clear or light-coloured fluid. Depending on area of skin involved, horse may be tender in local areas – reluctant to move – generally in pain – in a state of shock if extensive areas involved.

Possible diagnosis: Burns – *see page 172*

# CHOKING

## ASSOCIATED SIGNS

► Distressed – refuses to eat – extends head and neck – salivates – coughs – grunts – paws the ground – agitation gives way to depression. Food and saliva may be regurgitated through nostrils – lump may be seen and felt on left side of neck.

Possible diagnosis: Choke – *see page 176*

# COUGH

Find below the group of associated signs that best fits what you observe in your horse.

BACKGROUND

According to the kind of disease, horses exhibit different kinds of cough. A soft, shallow cough may not catch your attention and so not alert you to the fact that something is wrong with the horse; a deep, moist, violent cough commands attention and urges you to do something about it. Don't be alarmed by the occasional cough as a horse feeding or nuzzling its bedding may be irritated by dust, a fine piece of chaff or straw. Regular or intermittent coughing should be investigated. Types of coughs include soft, shallow, deep, moist, dry, hacking, violent, and productive as in coughing up mucus or phlegm.

## ASSOCIATED SIGNS

► Obvious sign is horse bleeding from one or both nostrils after race, track work or sometimes swimming – bleeding may begin during exercise, immediately after, or sometimes hours after exercise has finished – blood may lie inside nostrils, drip to ground, or flow freely. Some horses bleed in the lungs – only signs of this may be laboured breathing, distress and coughing – often the more serious type of haemorrhage.

Possible diagnosis: Bleeder (Epistaxis) – *see page 164*

---

► Clear watery discharge from both nostrils – persistent hacking cough – clear watery discharge from eyes – may be normal between bouts of coughing attacks.

Possible diagnosis: Bronchial Asthma – *see page 170*

---

► Distressed – refuses to eat – extends head and neck – salivates – coughs – grunts – paws the ground – agitation gives way to depression. Food and saliva may be regurgitated through nostrils – lump may be seen and felt on left side of neck.

Possible diagnosis: Choke – *see page 176*

---

► Dry cough – discharge from both nostrils – initially clear and watery – progressing to thick mucus – temperature – loss of appetite – lethargy.

Possible diagnosis: Equine Influenza – *see page 201*

---

► Incubation period of infection about 2 weeks – symptoms of a cold – temperature up – nasal discharge – sneezing – respiratory disease – abortion may occur up to 4 months after infection when mare appears healthy – abortion usually occurs from 5th month onwards. Foetus expelled rapidly with placenta – virus can affect brain and spinal cord of mare causing paralysis of hindquarters – foetus aborted after 6 months shows discolouration of placental fluid and hooves due to diarrhoea in uterus. Disease found throughout world including Australia.

Possible diagnosis: Equine Viral Rhinopneumonitis (Equine Herpes Virus I) – *see page 202*

---

► Young foals with purulent discharge from both nostrils – rattling sound in chest – laboured breathing – often stimulated by handling – harsh coat – elevated temperature.

Possible diagnosis: Foal Pneumonia (Rattles) – *see page 204*

---

► Nasal discharge – weight loss – rapid, shallow breathing – hear moisture in chest – ulcerations of nasal cavity and skin – often erupting on inside of hock – nodules under skin are up to 2 cm in diameter and discharge a honey-like pus.

Possible diagnosis: Glanders – *see page 216*

---

► Weight loss – dull harsh coat – pot belly – pale mucous membranes of eyelids and gums – diarrhoea – tail rubbing – poor appetite – reduced performance – poor stamina – colic – coughing in young foals – botfly eggs on coat.

Possible diagnosis: Parasites (in foals) – *see page 248*

---

► Sudden onset – temperature – not eating – lethargic – rapid shallow respiration – stands rather than lies down – doesn't want to move or turn round – short shallow cough. If you listen to chest with your ear you may hear a dry rasping sound. Tapping chest with your fingers may reveal a horizontal line of dullness – level of horizontal line varies depending on volume of fluid produced by pleura (lining of chest) – if you listen to chest below horizontal line, respiratory sounds are dull or non-existent – swelling may appear under chest and in lower limbs. Death is not uncommon 2–3 weeks after onset of symptoms.

Possible diagnosis: Pleurisy – *see page 260*

---

► Discharge from both nostrils – off food – lethargic – rapid shallow respiration – high temperature – breath may have foul odour – hear moisture in chest as horse breathes in and out – doesn't want to move or lie down – nostrils may be flared.

Possible diagnosis: Pneumonia – *see page 261*

---

► Copious, purulent discharge from both nostrils – loss of appetite – slight cough – lymph nodes under jaw inflamed and swollen – temperature – laboured respiration.

Possible diagnosis: Strangles – *see page 283*

# DRY, BROKEN HOOF

## ASSOCIATED SIGNS

► Dry hooves – cracks – pieces of wall breaking away.

Possible diagnosis: Brittle Hooves – *see page 169*

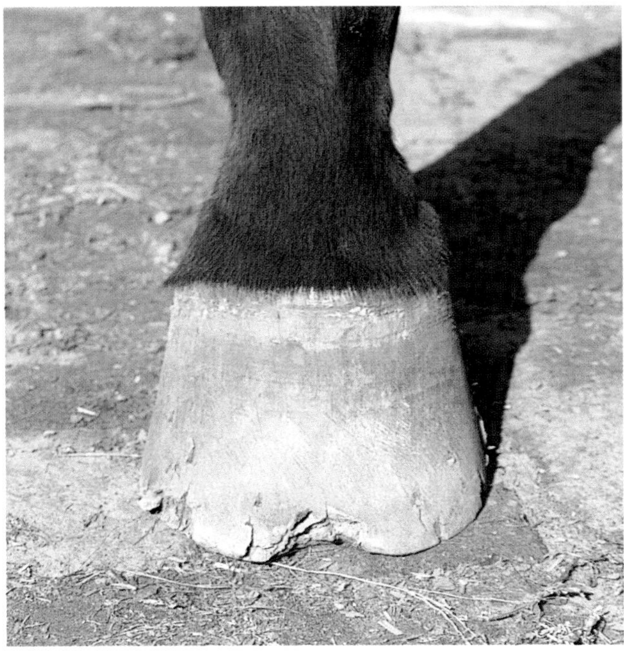

Brittle hoof

# DUNG EATING

## ASSOCIATED SIGNS

- Horse eating dung – suspicion aroused when mucking out stable or yard – little or no dung found – keep in mind horse may be constipated.

Possible diagnosis: Depraved Appetite – *see page 195*

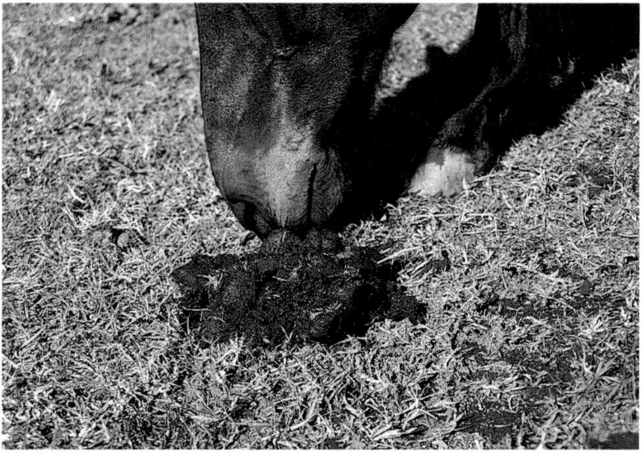

Depraved appetite — dung eating

# EAR PROBLEMS

Find below the group of associated signs that best fits what you observe in your horse.

## ASSOCIATED SIGNS

► One or both ears tend to droop – horse very sensitive to ears being touched or putting on bridle – rubbing ears – shaking head – holding head on one side – dark wax discharge from ear.

Possible diagnosis:
Ear Mites
*– see page 198*

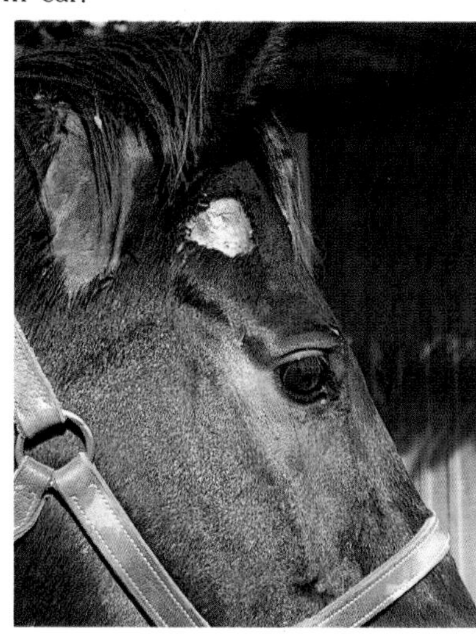

Hair loss from rubbing due to mites inside the ear canal

► Horse rubbing ear – shaking head – affected ear droops (not erect) – sensitive to putting on bridle – head may tilt to affected side – ear very sensitive to touch – may be odour and purulent fluid discharge.

Possible diagnosis:
Otitis Externa
*– see page 246*

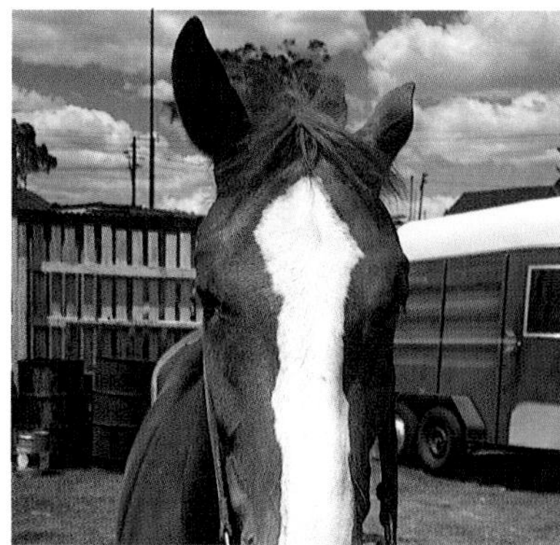

Otitis externa: the affected ear droops

# EYE PROBLEMS

Find below the group of associated signs that best fits what you observe in your horse.

## ASSOCIATED SIGNS

► Lens is partly or wholly cloudy – one or both eyes may be involved – some sight may be present. If lens is

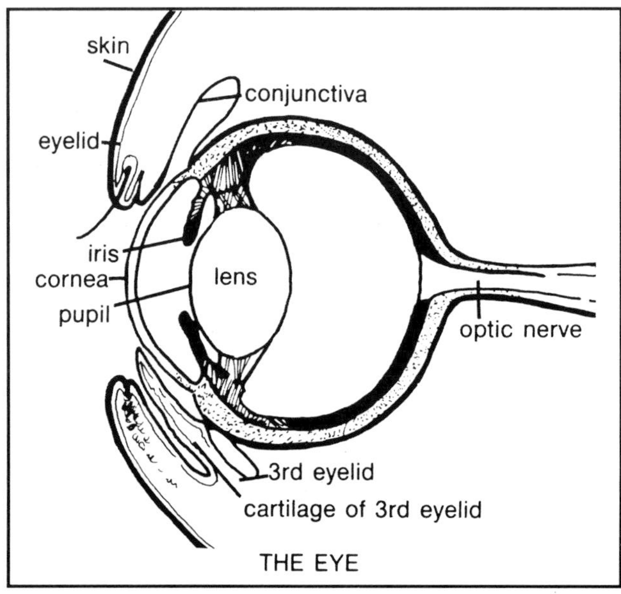


THE EYE

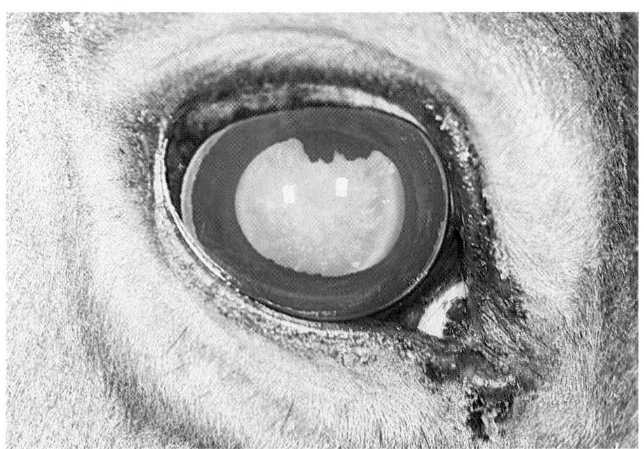

Cataract: the lens is cloudy

dense and silvery white – pupil usually dilated – total blindness in that eye. If horse totally blind in both eyes – will walk into walls and other objects – often subjects itself to severe abrasions. If horse totally blind in one eye often walks into objects on that side – when approached on blind side will often jump with fright when touched. If horse partially blind in one or both eyes may shy or balk at objects unnecessarily – may have difficulty in negotiating objects when light is subdued, as it is at dusk.

Possible diagnosis: Cataract – *see page 175*

---

► Conjunctival membrane very red, swollen and moist – discharge varies from copious amounts of clear watery fluid that runs down cheek to thick yellow-green pus that lies in corner of eyelids, sometimes matting them together – one or both eyes may be involved.

Possible diagnosis: Conjunctivitis – *see page 182*

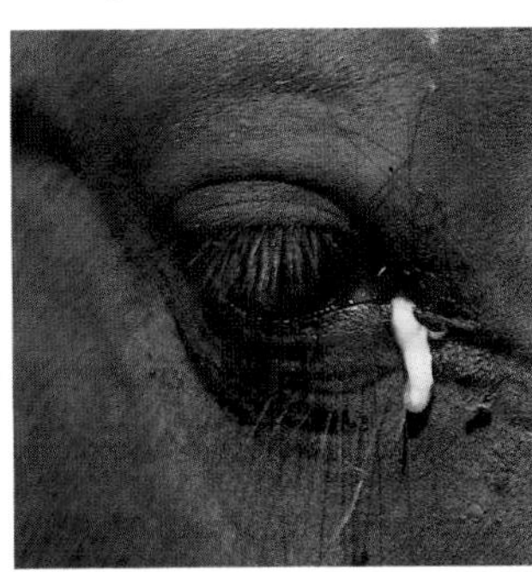

Discharge of yellow-green pus is a sign of conjunctivitis

► Tears streaming down cheek – eyelid(s) partially or completely closed – appearance of cornea or surface of

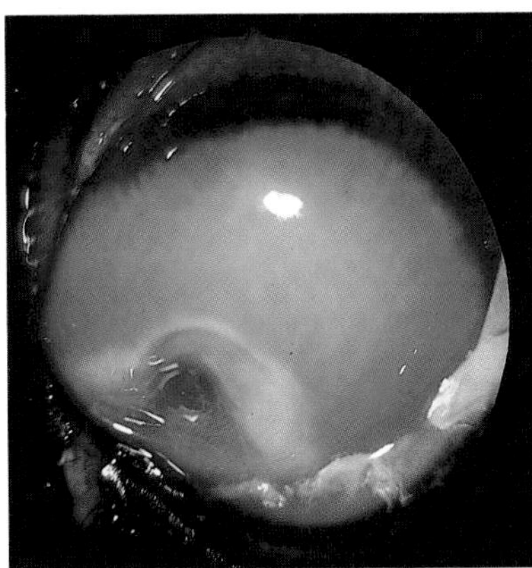

A deep corneal ulcer

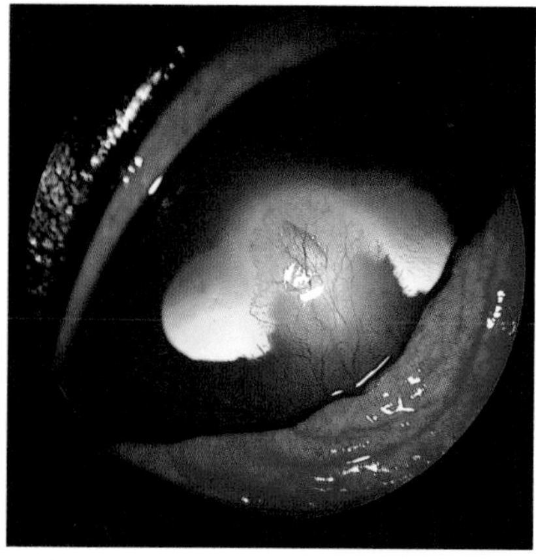

The cornea has a cloudy surface (keratitis) with a corneal ulcer in the centre

affected eye can vary from dull and hazy in small area to whole corneal surface being opaque and bluish-white in colour – a small pit, varying in depth, may be seen if cornea is ulcerated – scar formation following ulceration is common.

Possible diagnosis: Corneal Ulcer; Keratitis – *see page 188*

---

► Weeping of affected eye – evidenced by continual wet patch below it – partial closure of eyelid of affected eye or rubbing eye to alleviate constant irritation – closer examination reveals upper and/or lower eyelid turns in, causing eyelashes to rub on surface of eyeball (cornea), thus irritating it.

Possible diagnosis: Entropion – *see page 198*

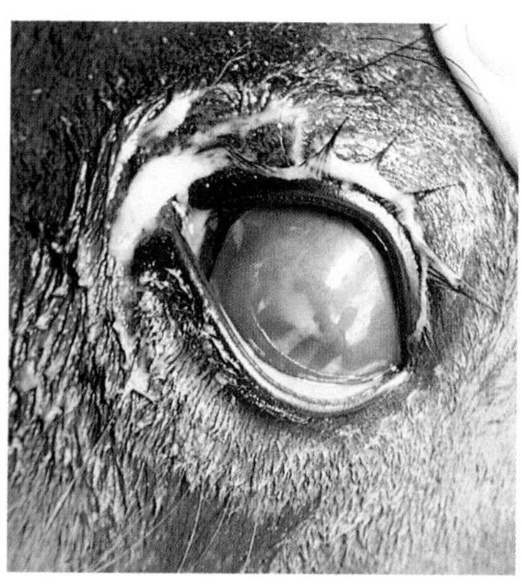

Entropion

► Tears running down cheeks – sensitivity to light – closing of eyelids – conjunctivitis – pus may be seen behind cornea – pupil sometimes unable to dilate. Generally affects horses 3–7 years of age – may clear up or improve then recur 3–12 months later – may affect one or both eyes.

Possible diagnosis: Recurrent Uveitis (Periodic Ophthalmia) – *see page 270*

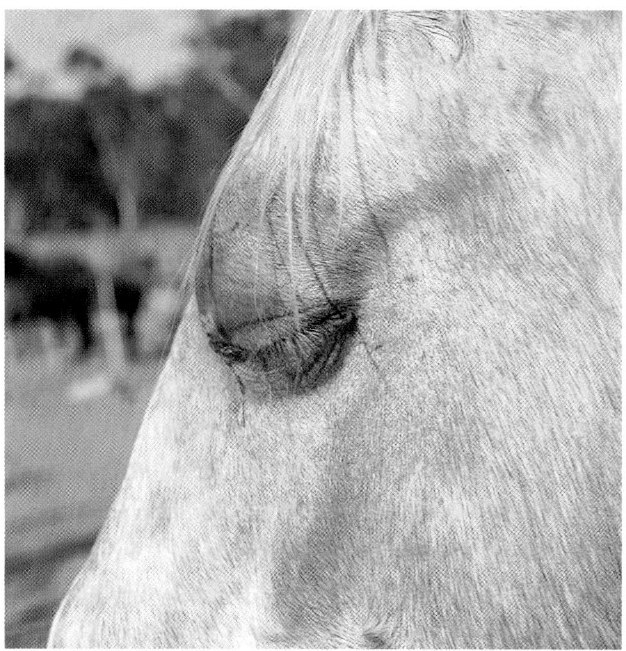

Eyelids closed — sensitivity to light with recurrent uveitis

# FOAL DISEASES & PROBLEMS

Find below the group of associated signs that best fits what you observe in your horse.

## ASSOCIATED SIGNS

► Foal cannot pass motion – signs of straining – appears constipated – becomes colicky – no anal opening – abdominal pain.

Possible diagnosis: Atresia Ani – *see page 159*

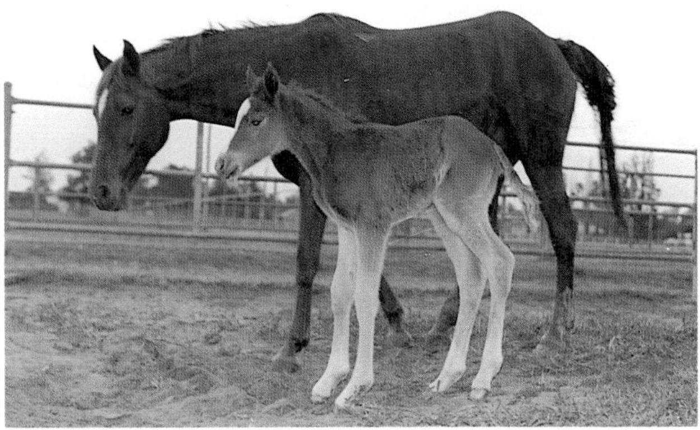

Foal straining: constipation

► Foal strains without results – often observed 12–18 hours after birth – throws itself to ground and thrashes violently.

Possible diagnosis: Constipation – *see page 183*

---

► Foal stands on its toes or even knuckles over and walks on front of fetlock.

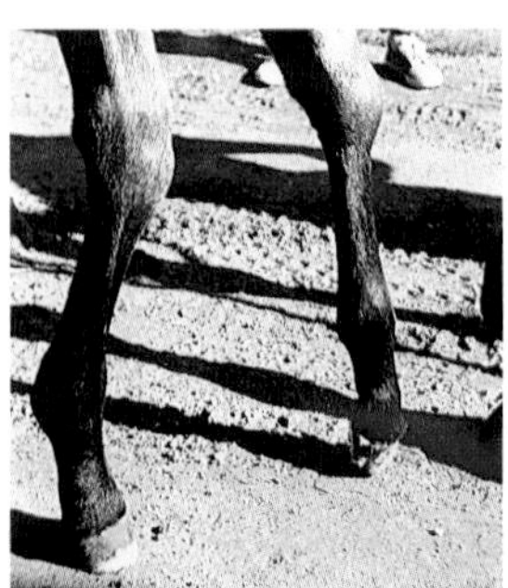

Possible diagnosis: Contracted Tendons – *see page 186*

Contracted tendons

► Dung is fluid, putrid. Foal strains – tucks up abdomen. Can cause death.

Possible diagnosis: Diarrhoea – *see page 196*

---

► Weeping of affected eye – evidenced by continual wet patch below it – partial closure of eyelid of affected eye or rubbing eye to alleviate constant irritation – closer examination reveals upper and/or lower eyelid turns in, causing eyelashes to rub on surface of eyeball (cornea), thus irritating it.

Possible diagnosis: Entropion – *see page 198*

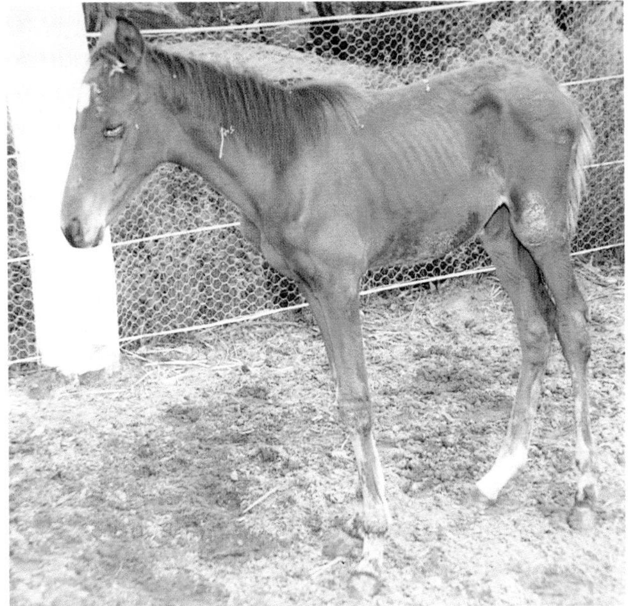

This foal has pneumonia

► Young foals with purulent discharge from both nostrils – rattling sound in chest – coughing – laboured breathing – often stimulated by handling – harsh coat – elevated temperature.

Possible diagnosis: Foal Pneumonia (Rattles) – *see page 204*

---

► Found in new-born foal – sluggish – dull – weak – no longer suckles – lies down – rapid shallow breathing (panting), especially after exercise – anaemic (pale gums and conjunctiva) – then gums and conjunctiva change to varying shades of yellow – after 24 hours urine dark brown in colour – may collapse.

Possible diagnosis: Isoimmune Haemolytic Jaundice – *see page 228*

---

► Heat, pain and swelling in affected joint(s) of new-born foal – lameness – stiffness in movement – temperature rise.

Possible diagnosis: Joint ill – *see page 229*

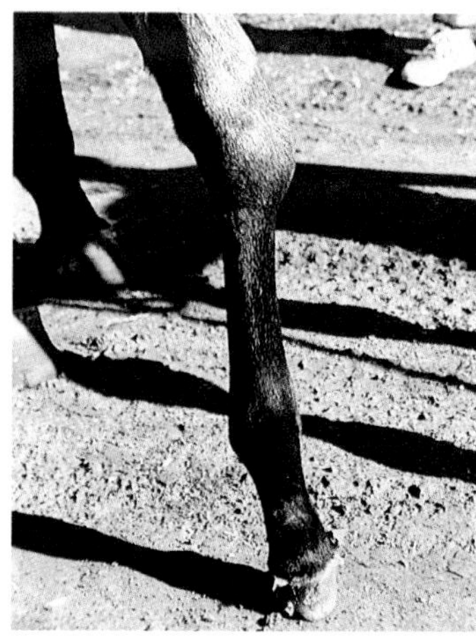

Joint ill

► Young foals with knee(s) bowing inwards.

Possible diagnosis: Knock Knees – *see page 230*

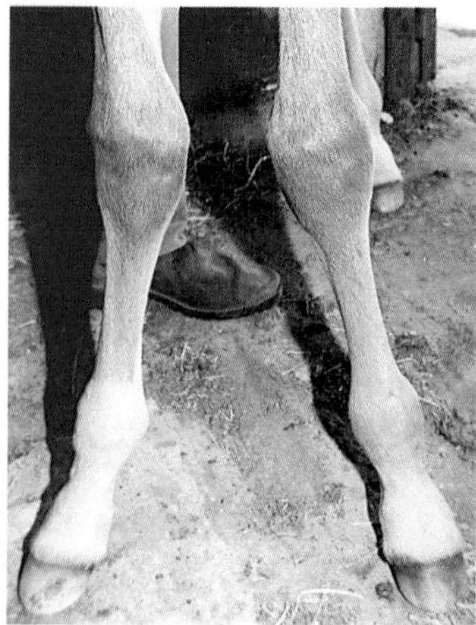

Knock knees

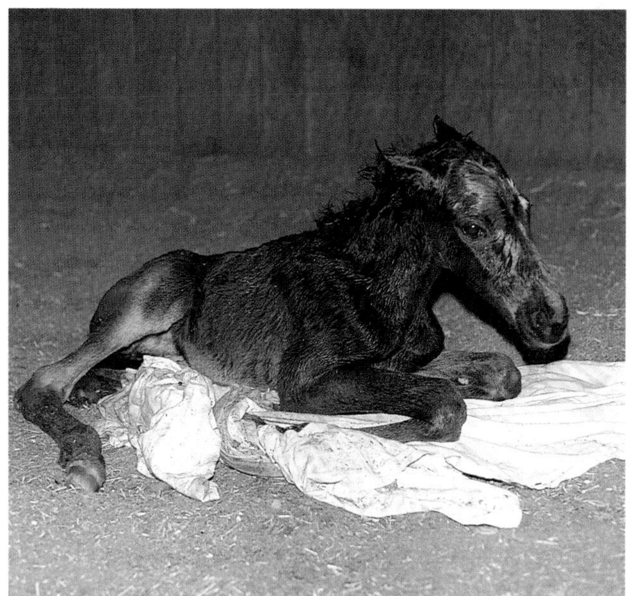

An orphan foal

► When foal loses its mother at birth or shortly after – also foal whose mother, for some reason, has no milk or cannot nurse her offspring.

Possible diagnosis: Orphan Foal – *see page 244*

---

► Urine drips from stump of navel cord – flow increases when foal strains to urinate – often wet patch around umbilical stump – occurs in new-born foal.

Possible diagnosis: Patent Urachus – *see page 258*

---

► Foal born after spending less than 330 days in uterus – mare's gestation period on average is 342 days (can be 10 days more or less).

Possible diagnosis: Premature Foal – *see page 264*

---

► Foal shows signs of depression 12–24 hours after birth – strains repeatedly to urinate – very little or no urine passed – straining can be similar in constipated foal – do not confuse.

Possible diagnosis: Ruptured Bladder – *see page 273*

► Foal very depressed – weak – fails to suckle – breathes rapidly – lies down – harsh coat – initially high temperature that falls and becomes sub-normal as foal deteriorates – foal may die suddenly.

Possible diagnosis: Septicaemia (Blood Poisoning) – *see page 277*

---

► Swelling in region of navel – may be up to 5 cm in diameter.

Possible diagnosis: Umbilical Hernia – *see page 293*

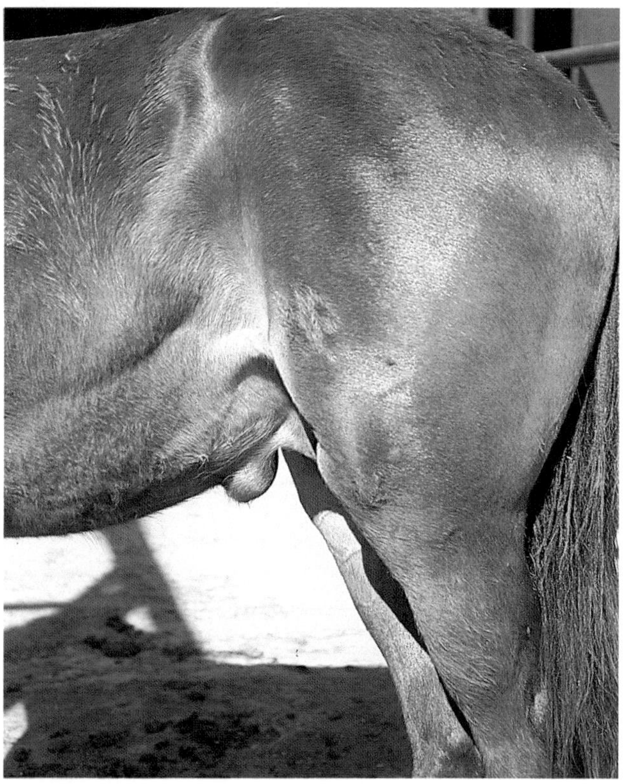

Umbilical (navel) hernia

► Foal walks on back of fetlock joint.

Possible diagnosis: Weak Flexor Tendons – *see page 296*

# FOALING & BIRTH DIFFICULTIES

Find below the group of associated signs that best fits what you observe in your horse.

## ASSOCIATED SIGNS

► Mare straining in labour – obvious contractions – after about 25 minutes no foal appears.

After 15 minutes of obvious straining and contractions, mare appears to give up – in following half-hour her efforts are weak and less frequent.

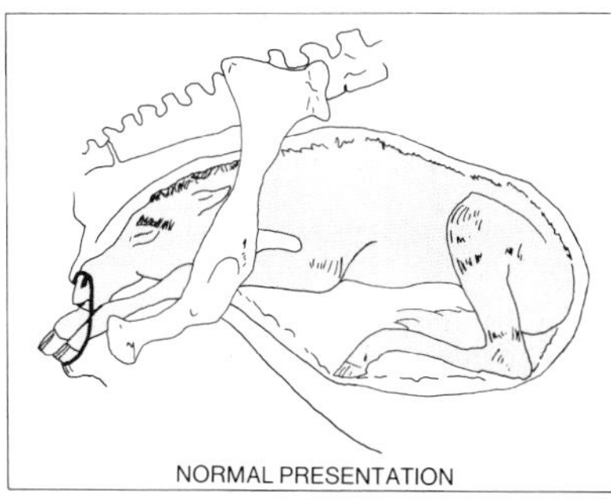

NORMAL PRESENTATION

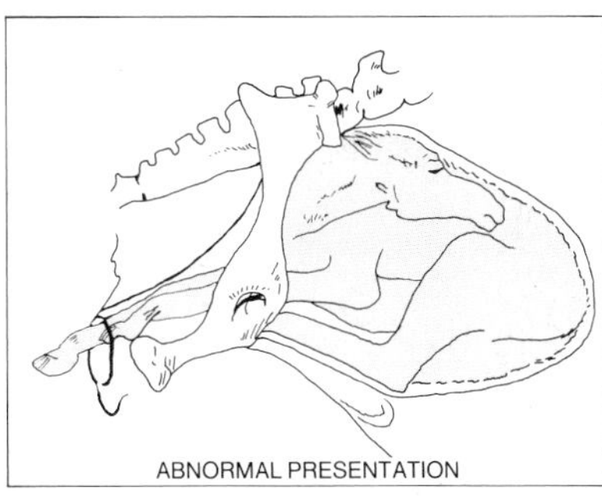

ABNORMAL PRESENTATION

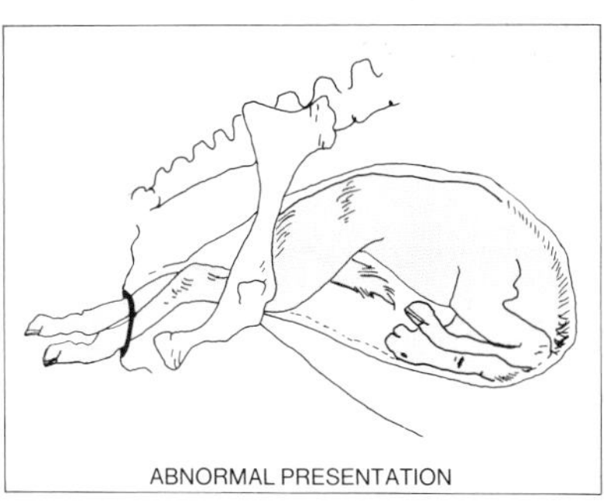

ABNORMAL PRESENTATION

No obvious contractions – mare continually gets up and down – shows signs of pain by kicking, swishing her tail, looking at flanks.

Other signs are one leg of foal presented – excessive bulging of mare's anus – forefeet presented but head turned back in uterus – foal lying on back with soles of feet and lower jaw upper-most – foal doubled on itself so head, forefeet, hind feet all presented together – hind feet presented first with soles facing upwards – buttocks and tail of foal presented (breech) – buttocks, tail, points of both hocks presented – twin foals.

Possible diagnosis: Birth Difficulties – *see page 163*

---

► Mare's abdomen large and swollen – sweating – restless – agitated – pawing ground – stretching – swishing tail – lying down – getting up – fluid from vagina – straining – foetal membrane appears at vagina.

Possible diagnosis: Foaling – *see page 205*

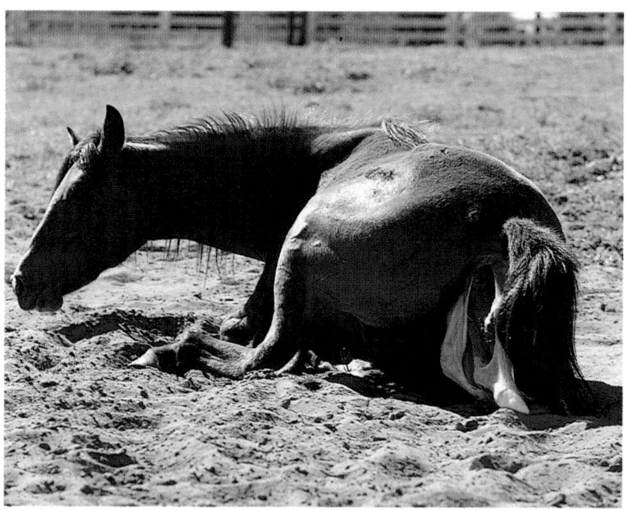

The foetal membranes appear at the vagina

# GAIT ABNORMALITY

Find below the group of associated signs that best fits what you observe in your horse.

## BACKGROUND

Gait abnormalities are as varied as the causes. Some are brought on by an unskilled or unbalanced rider, others by ill-fitting or badly adjusted tack. Some are due to poor conformation, poor co-ordination, or poor hoof trimming and/or shoeing; others are related to the horse's individual action ('way of going').

Many gait abnormalities can be improved or eradicated by corrective trimming and shoeing. Before attempting to do so, examine the horse carefully in regard to conformation, stance, relationship of pastern to hoof, type of feet, position of frog in relation to ground, abnormal wear and action. Trimming the hoof to correct a conformation fault or abnormal gait should be done carefully. Don't try to correct the problem by severely trimming the hoof at the first attempt, do it little by little. The only tools required are a tang rasp and a pair of hoof nippers.

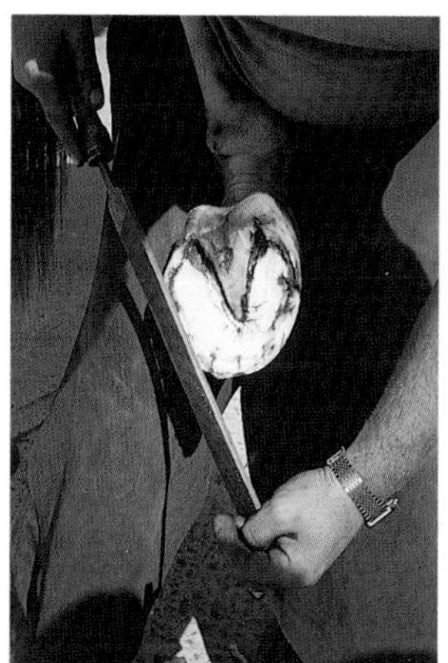

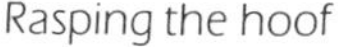

Rasping the hoof

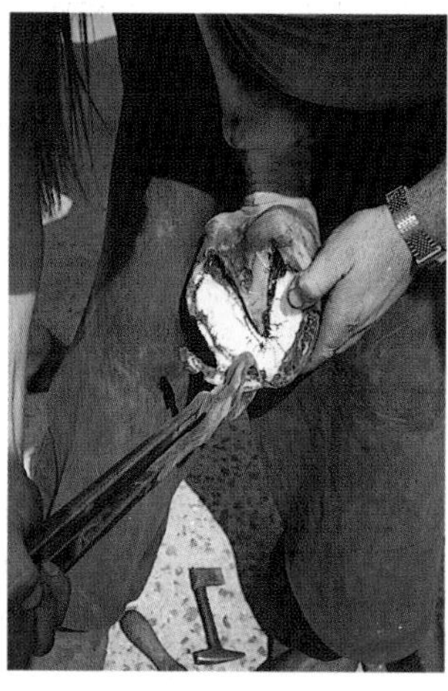

The hoof wall being trimmed with hoof nippers

Horses that continue to give trouble after corrective shoeing and trimming often respond to the treatment of allowing the feet to grow then being worked on a hard, smooth, level surface. This allows the feet to be worn naturally, helping them to find their own natural level. When this is achieved, the horse may be shod.

## ASSOCIATED SIGNS

► Inside edge of foot in motion touches inside of fetlock of opposite leg – may occur with forelegs or hind legs.

Possible diagnosis: Brushing – *see page 171*

---

► Heels of the hoof close together, often with deep furrow between them – frog may be small, hard with shrivelled appearance and not in contact with ground – sole often much more concave than normal – horse may or may not be lame – condition more common in front feet, either one or both.

Possible diagnosis: Contracted Heels – *see page 185*

---

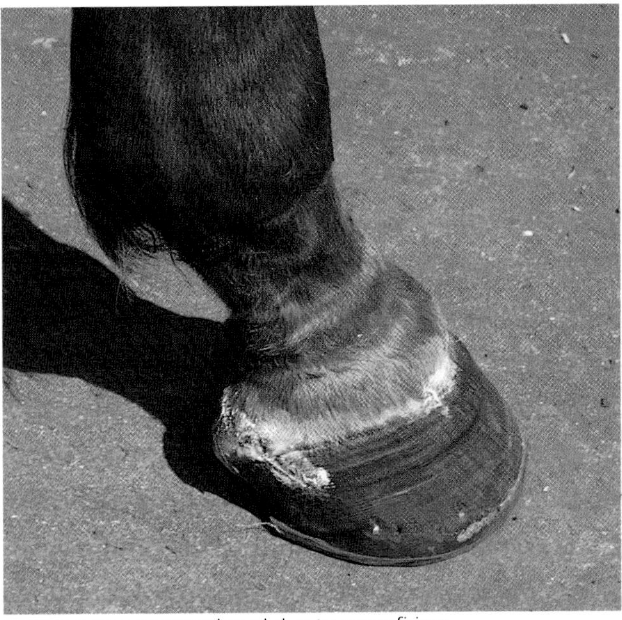

Wound on coronary band due to cross firing

► Toe or inside wall of hind foot strikes inside quarter of opposite forefoot – breaks skin, often causing deep wound.

Possible diagnosis: Cross Firing – *see page 190*

---

► When cantering or galloping, back of fetlock of hind limbs touches ground, grazing skin, sometimes severely.

Possible diagnosis: Getting Down Behind (Getting down on the Bumpers) – *see page 215*

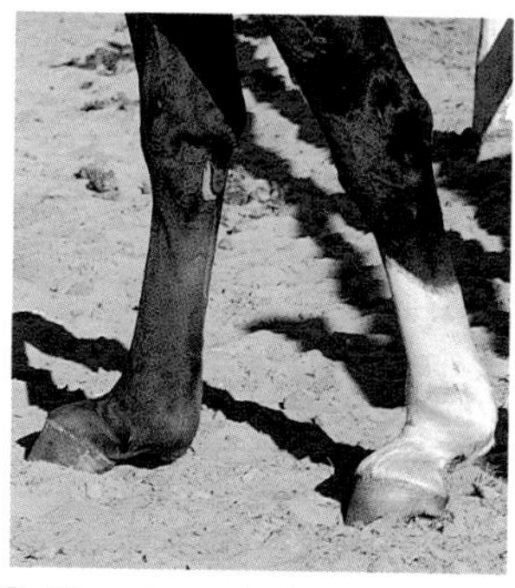

Getting down behind — the back of the fetlock is touching the ground

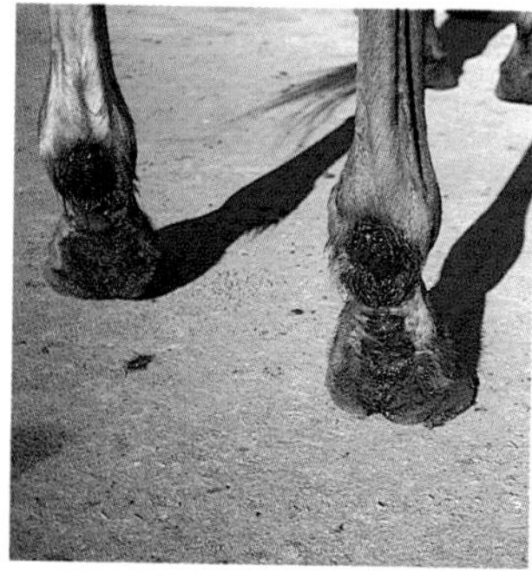

Going down on the bumpers

---

► Hind foot steps on heel of forefoot on same side – often toe of hind foot steps on heel of shoe on forefoot, pulling it off.

Possible diagnosis: Over-Reaching (Forging) – *see page 247*

# HEATSTROKE

## ASSOCIATED SIGNS

► Sudden onset following hard work in hot, humid weather conditions, confinement in stables with poor ventilation, crowding in yards or floats with other horses. Mucous membranes brick red – rapid respiration – dilated nostrils – heart rate rapid – patchy sweating – high temperature – staggers – collapse – unable to get up – convulsions – in some cases death.

Possible diagnosis: Heatstroke – *see page 222*

# INFECTED PENIS

## ASSOCIATED SIGNS

- Creamy discharge from prepuce (sheath) – irritation is indicated by rubbing or dropping out of penis – when penis is extended surface is covered with heavy, waxy scales – the folds are inflamed and swollen and have an accumulation of pus – unpleasant odour associated with discharge.

Possible diagnosis: Infected Penis and Prepuce – *see page 225*

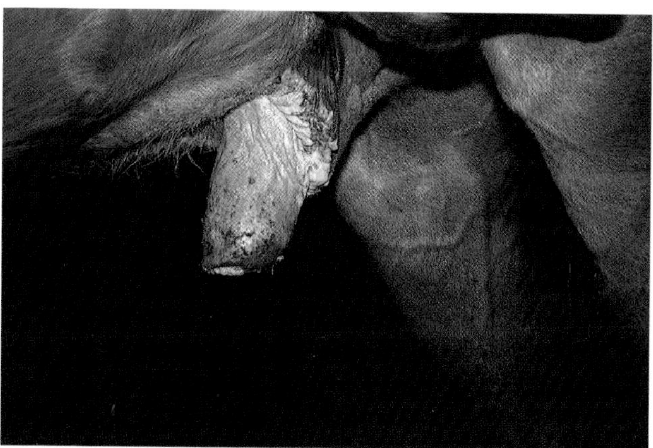

Infected penis and prepuce

# LAMENESS

Find below the group of associated signs that best fits what you observe in your horse.

## BACKGROUND

Lameness can render a horse useless or cause it to perform below its normal level of efficiency. Lameness is generally the result of soreness in a limb, that the horse will then favour, or of reduced flexibility in a joint, whereby the horse's ability to stretch out is restricted. Lameness in most horses is obvious, but in some cases the observer needs a certain expertise to make a correct judgement.

In most cases, lameness is located in the forelimbs because they bear 60–65% of the horse's weight as well as providing some force to assist the hind limbs in propelling the horse forward. Lameness is usually concentrated in that section of the leg between foot and knee – hip and shoulder problems rarely cause lameness.

Contributing causes of lameness are injury, infection, poor nutrition (calcium imbalance), inherited defects and disorders of nervous and circulatory systems. Signs of lameness vary markedly: lameness is acute when the horse cannot put its foot to the ground; sub-acute when the horse uses its leg but has a distinct limp; chronic if the horse is vaguely lame, if its lameness is intermittent or if it has been going on for a long time. Sometimes a horse is lame when it first walks out of the stable but then the lameness disappears, or only comes on after work. Other signs associated with lameness are inflammation, heat, swelling and pain on palpation. The location and causes of some types of lameness are readily detected, e.g. there may be a nail puncture in the sole of the foot.

When examining a horse for lameness, first check it in the stable. Look at it as it stands squarely and motionless. Check to see if it is bearing its full weight on all four legs, if it has any swellings or if there are signs of injury such as cuts, bruises or grazes.

Ask a handler to lead the horse out of the stable so that you can examine it in motion on a hard, even surface, preferably concrete or asphalt. The handler should look straight ahead, not at the horse, so that the horse is led freely and without any interference to its straight forward movement and head action.

Ask the handler to walk the horse away from you in a straight line for 25 metres, then turn it sharply to the left (near side) and walk it back straight towards you. Step aside to allow it to pass and observe it from the side. Continue to watch the horse walking for 25 metres, then ask the handler to turn it sharply to the right (off side) and bring it back, past you. The same procedures are repeated at the trot, in a circle, first one way then the other, with you standing in the centre.

Keep an eye on the horse's head because, when the horse steps on its lame leg, the head goes up to help take some of the weight off it. Correspondingly, the head goes down when the good leg takes the weight, a phenomenon often called 'head nod associated with lameness'.

If the horse is lame in both front or both back legs, it will have a stilted, proppy action.

The length of stride may be shorter in the lame leg, an action call 'stepping short'.

If observing the horse at walk or trot, and the lameness is obscure and difficult to isolate, it can often be made more apparent by placing a rider on the horse's back.

If the observer listens carefully to the sound made by the horse's hooves on a hard surface such as concrete or asphalt, an irregularity in rhythm may indicate lameness.

Lameness can sometimes be detected by palpation. Start at the foot, feeling with your hand to detect heat, then tap gently with a hammer in various spots to detect pain. If lameness involves the foot, remove shoe, check nails and nail holes and clean foot thoroughly, looking for puncture wounds, bruising, corns and cracks. Feel the leg, particularly the joints, for swelling and heat; press, squeeze, bend, testing for pain and flexibility.

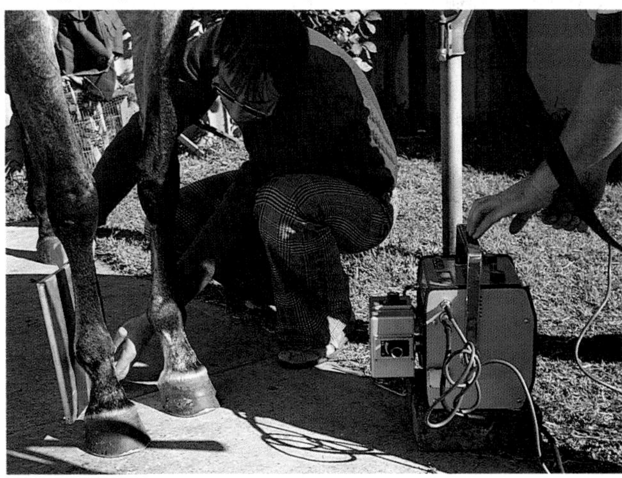

Taking a leg X-ray

To treat lameness that cannot be simply rectified, call your veterinarian. He has a detailed knowledge of the anatomy and physiology of the horse and has probably treated other similar cases. He is also experienced in the technology of X-ray, hoof testing and nerve blocks.

You can help the veterinarian by preparing a well-organised history of the horse. Include such matters as when it was last shod, when it was last ridden and how hard, what kind of surface it was ridden on, when it became lame (before, during or immediately after exercise, or the next day).

The veterinarian should be called when the horse is lame, not after a week's rest when the horse is sound. Don't call him if the horse has been treated with anti-inflammatory drugs as they mask lameness and make the task of diagnosis more difficult. If you are uncertain which leg is lame, don't pretend that you know and tell the veterinarian that it is the right foreleg – he will waste time checking, when all the time the lameness may be in the near side hind leg.

## ASSOCIATED SIGNS

► Swelling localised in joint(s) – in initial stage (acute) may be firm, warm, swollen, painful to touch – with time (chronic stage) becomes hard – often not warm to touch – less painful – may restrict movement of joint – eventually permanent joint damage.

Possible diagnosis: Arthritis – *see page 159*

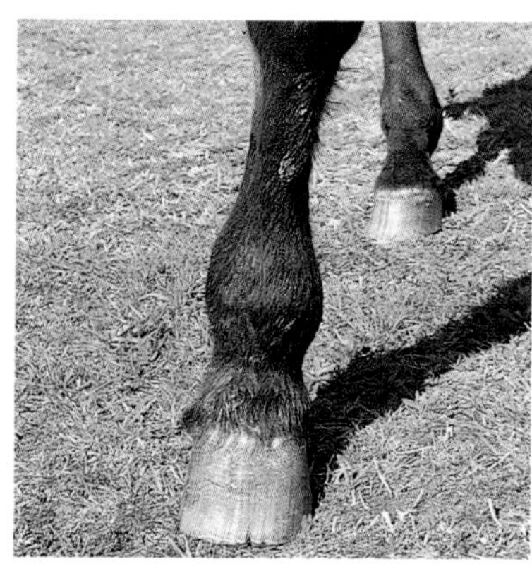

Arthritis: swollen fetlock joint

► Soft fluid-filled swelling on upper and inner side of hock – more often than not, no heat or pain associated with swelling – lameness, if present, is of a mild temporary nature.

Possible diagnosis: Bog Spavin – *see page 165*

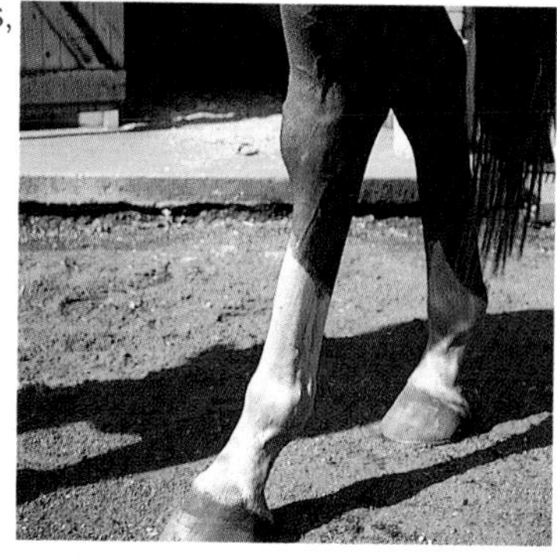

Bog spavin: a soft swelling on the upper inner side of the hock

► Hard bony enlargement felt and seen on lower and inner side of hock – horse lame when cold – lameness characterised by reduced flexion of hock and shortening of stride in affected leg – often disappears as horse warms up with exercise – sometimes worsens.

Possible diagnosis: Bone Spavin – *see page 166*

---

► Swelling in any one of the legs (mainly a front leg) behind cannon bone, running from knee to fetlock. In early stages: swelling – heat – pain on pressure – may step short or be severely lame – in later stages, swelling reduced and localised leaving hard fibrous bow in tendon.

Possible diagnosis: Bowed Tendon – *see page 167*

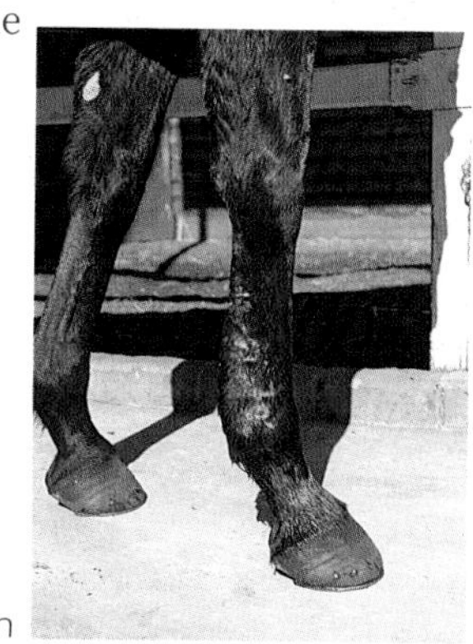

Bowed tendon

---

► If you clean sole with a hoof knife, bruising will be evident by presence of blood under the surface – if bruising severe, horse will show signs of lameness and react to pressure on sole.

Possible diagnosis: Bruised Sole – *see page 170*

---

► Round, soft, fluid-filled swelling on point of elbow – up to 10 cm in diameter – most cases not sore to touch – lameness slight and temporary.

Possible diagnosis: Capped Elbow – *see page 173*

---

► Swelling on point of hock – in early stages round, soft, fluid-filled, up to 10 cm in diameter – not sore to touch – lameness, if present, is slight and temporary. Old swellings filled with fibrous tissue – hard to touch.

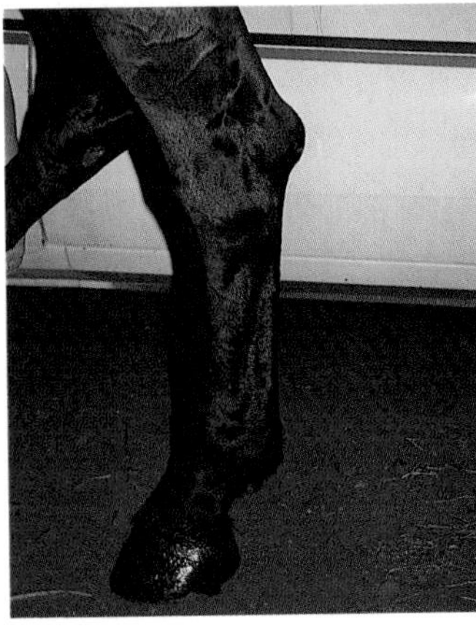

Possible diagnosis: Capped Hock – *see page 174*

Capped hock: soft, fluid-filled swelling on the point of the hock

---

► Swelling in localised circumscribed area of knee or more generalised – recent swellings soft – older swellings may be very hard – flexibility of knee restricted – signs of pain when knee bent.

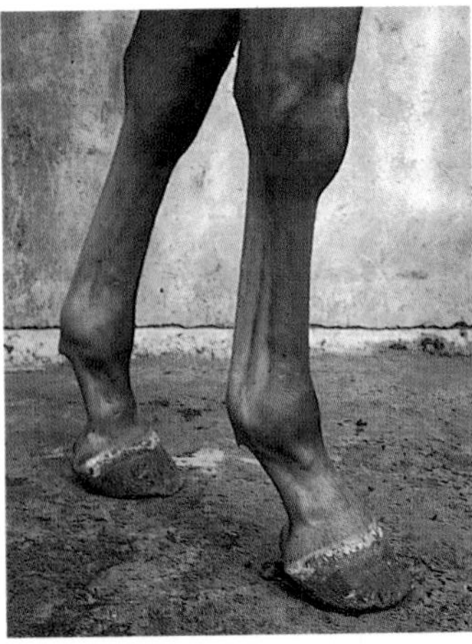

Possible diagnosis: Carpitis – *see page 175*

Carpitis: general swelling of the knee

► Collection of blood under sole in region of heel – horse shows signs of lameness.

Possible diagnosis: Corns – *see page 189*

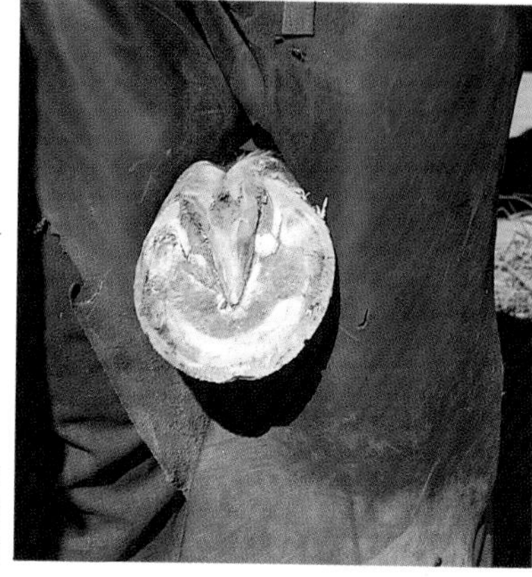

Sole cut away to expose blood (corn) in the region of the heel

---

► Swelling about 10 cm below point of hock – viewed from side semi-circular in shape – feels hard when pressed – if lameness present, it is only slight and temporary.

Possible diagnosis: Curb – *see page 191*

---

► Swelling 2.5 cm above knee – seen in yearlings and 2-year-olds when being broken in (educated) or trained – pain may be evident on palpation of swelling or flexion of knee – if lame, there is stilted, proppy action in affected leg.

Possible diagnosis: Epiphysitis – *see page 199*

---

► Horse reluctant to move – tends to lie down or change weight continually from one foot to another – if only front feet involved horse will stand with hind legs well up under body and its forelegs well forward – this position adopted so that as much weight as possible is taken off front feet – if forced to move horse will shuffle along, putting heels to ground first – affected feet are hot due to inflammation and increased arterial blood supply – throbbing of arteries running down either side of pastern can be felt with slight pressure of fingers.

Horse refuses to eat, sweats and trembles – symptoms reflect pain that horse is suffering – in severe cases its hoof or hooves may fall off – with chronic

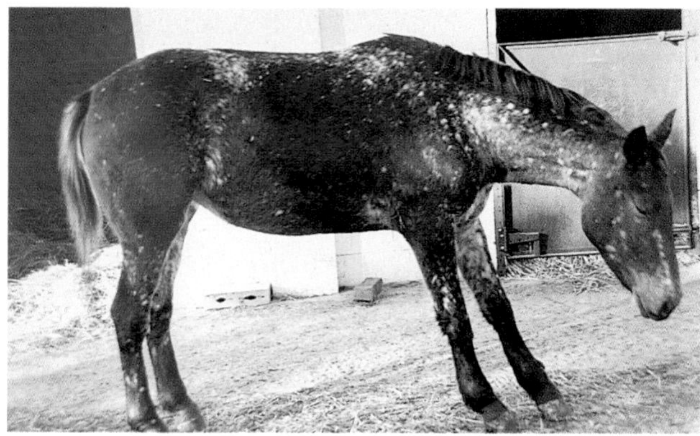

Trying to take the weight off its front feet — a classic position for a horse that has foundered

cases, horse intermittently lame putting heels of affected feet to ground first – feet are often warm – sole dropped and convex instead of being concave – ring-like impressions are present on hoof wall.

Possible diagnosis: Founder (Laminitis) – *see page 211*

---

► One or more of following signs may be evident: lameness – swelling – pain – haemorrhage – anxiety – sweating – trembling – limb hanging limply or bone protruding.

Possible diagnosis: Fracture – *see page 212*

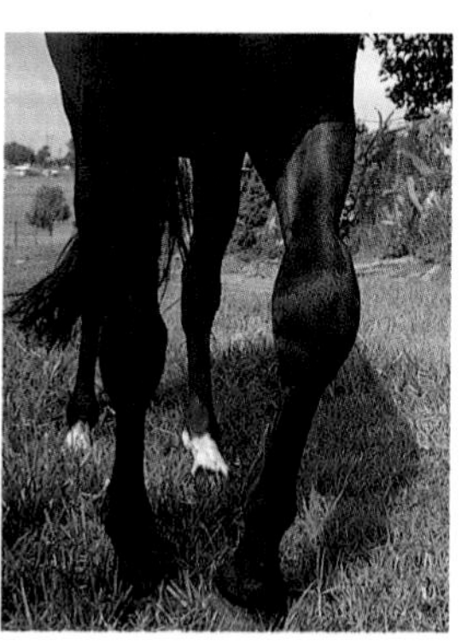

Fractured knee: horse cannot bear weight on leg

---

► Acute lameness, usually in one front leg, immediately horse pulls up from exercising – or may falter and stop during exercise – no sign of swelling or soreness in leg – severe pain exhibited when hoof testers (pincers) are applied to hoof or when hoof is tapped with a hammer – over number of days lameness does not improve.

Possible diagnosis: Fractured Pedal or Navicular Bone – *see page 258*

---

► Skin at back of pastern is inflamed – later becomes raw and bleeding – affected areas are sore to touch – hair may be lost – deep cracks with thickened skin on either side may develop – in severe cases swelling of pastern and fetlock accompany lameness.

Possible diagnosis
Greasy Heel
– *see page 216*

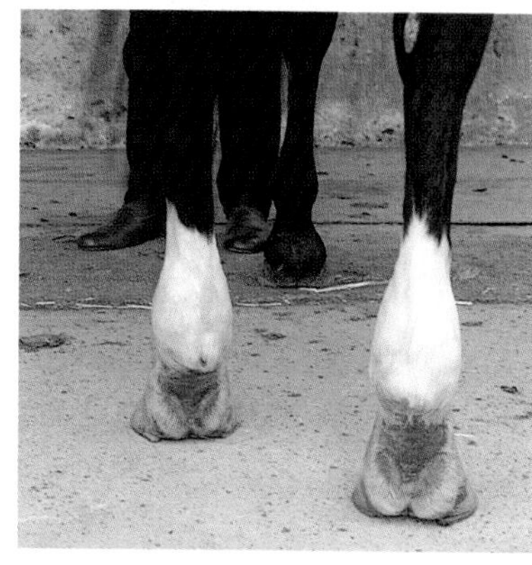

Greasy heel: inflamed skin lack of hair

---

► Crack in hoof wall varies from short and shallow to long and deep – crack can start at ground surface of hoof wall or at coronary band – if depth of crack involves sensitive tissues horse will probably be lame.

Possible diagnosis:
Hoof Crack
– *see page 223*

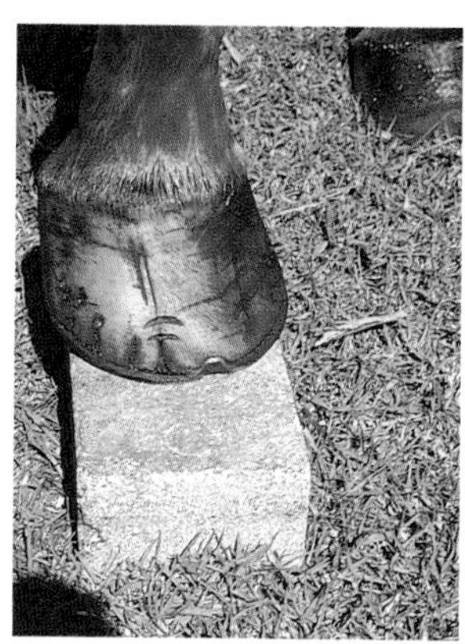

Crack running almost full length of the hoof wall

---

► Heat, pain and swelling in affected joint(s) of new-born foal – lameness – stiffness in movement – temperature rise.

Possible diagnosis: Joint ill – *see page 229*

---

- When stifle locked, hind leg assumes fully extended position with hoof bent backwards – when horse forced to move with stiff leg, front of hoof drags along ground – limb may remain locked in position of extension for hours or kneecap may be released every few steps, allowing leg to flex (bend) suddenly – often a snapping sound is heard as kneecap released – sudden release of kneecap with leg shooting forward can be mistaken for stringhalt (see page 284) by inexperienced observer.

Possible diagnosis: Locking of Stifle – *see page 237*

---

- Mild lameness shortly after shoeing – generally worsens each day – 3–7 days after being shod, horse is acutely lame, just touching ground with toe of foot – hoof wall is warm to touch – pastern may be swollen – arteries on either side of pastern supplying hoof pulsate more rapidly and strongly than normal. When squeezed with hoof testers (pincers) or tapped with hammer, severe pain exhibited by horse pulling foot away – pain is worse when pressure is applied over offending nail.

Possible diagnosis: Nail Prick – *see page 240*

---

- In early stages slight lameness that seems to fluctuate from one front foot to the other – as disease progresses horse steps short in both front legs, assuming a proppy, stilted gait, particularly at the trot – horse will often resent trotting and try to break into canter – when turning, rather than crossing its front legs, it will tend to shuffle around in order to lessen pressure on navicular bone.

Possible diagnosis: Navicular Disease – *see page 241*

---

- Swelling appears just above or below front of fetlock – usually hard – pain on bending fetlock and lameness are present.

Possible diagnosis: Osselets – *see page 245*

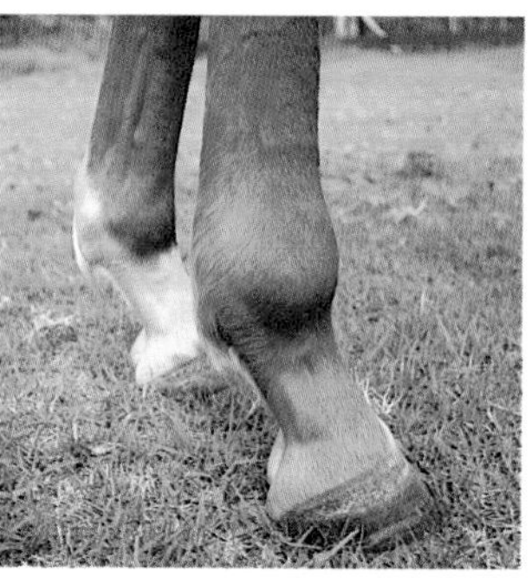

Osselets: a swelling just above the fetlock

► Lameness sometimes present in front feet – other times absent – often difficult to tell if in right front leg or left front leg – as condition progresses, lameness obvious in all gaits – characterised by a short step.

Possible diagnosis: Pedal Osteitis – *see page 259*

---

► Redness, swelling, heat and pain in region of heel and associated coronary band – discharge from small openings or cracks around coronary band – dry up and erupt again – fluctuating lameness associated with build-up of discharge.

Possible diagnosis: Quittor – *see page 266*

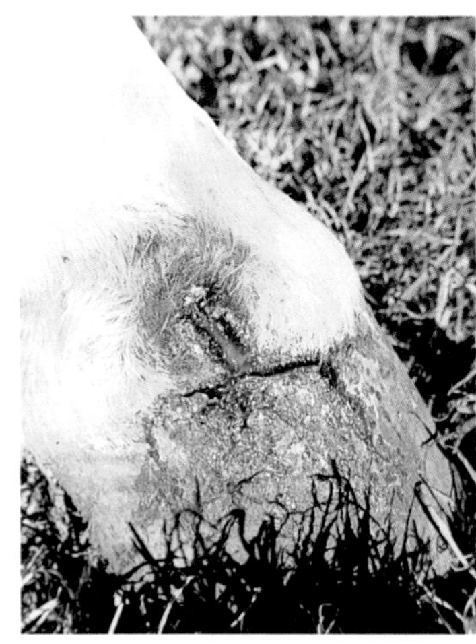

Quittor: discharge from a crack around the coronary band

---

► Swelling on front or sides of pastern – in early stages evidence of heat, swelling, pain on pressure, lameness

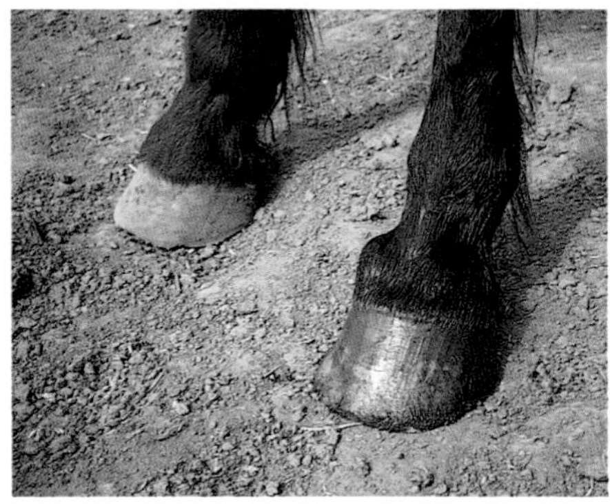

High ringbone

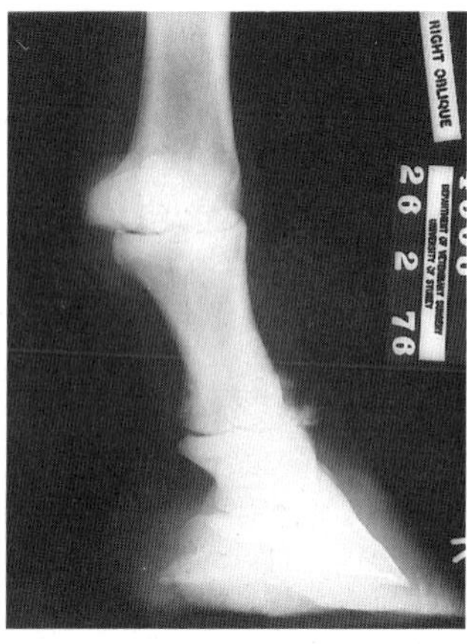


– in later stages bony swelling varying in size can be seen and felt on pastern.

Possible diagnosis: Ringbone – *see page 270*

X-ray showing high ringbone

---

► Separation of wall from sole at the toe – leaves a pocket or cavity running under wall – if hoof wall is tapped, it emits hollow sound – when shoe is removed and sole is pared back at toe, a hollow cavity is visible – often filled with black, foul-smelling, greasy, decaying hoof – horse may or may not be lame.

Possible diagnosis: Seedy Toe – *see page 276*

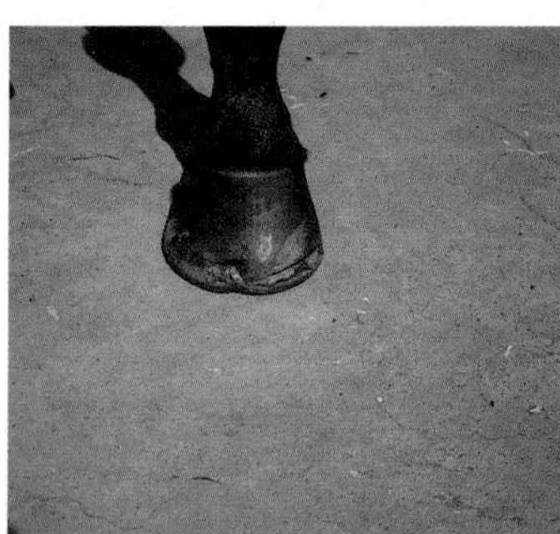

Seedy toe: separation of the hoof wall from the sole at the toe

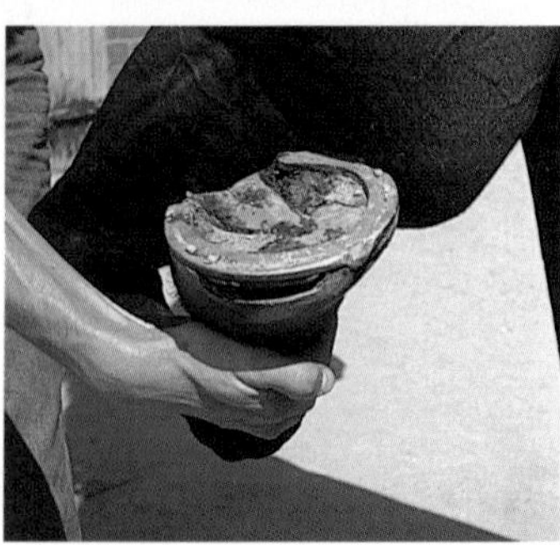

Seedy toe: a hollow cavity is visible under the hoof wall

► Swelling at back of fetlock – lameness – pain on application of pressure to sesamoid bones and on bending fetlock joint.

Possible diagnosis: Sesamoiditis – *see page 277*

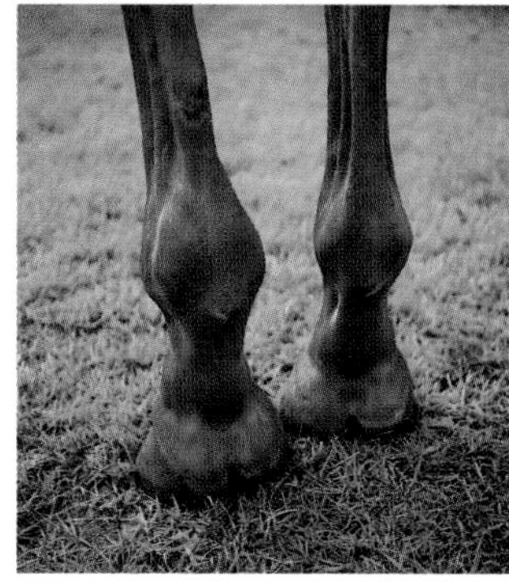

Sesamoiditis: swelling at the back of the fetlock

---

► Swelling on front of cannon bone – one or both limbs involved – warm and painful to touch – horse may show lameness or shortening of stride.

Possible diagnosis: Shin Soreness – *see page 278*

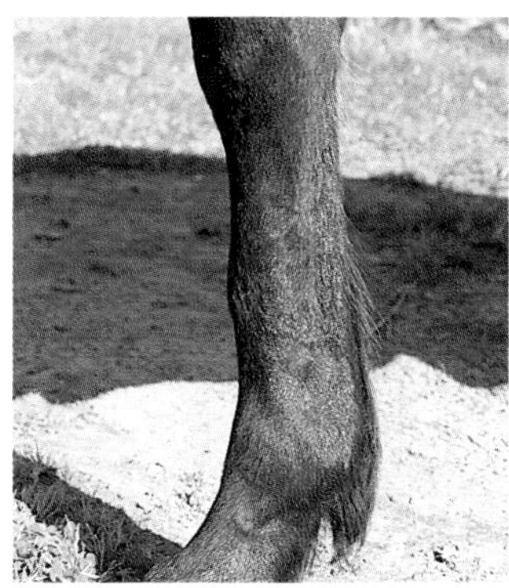

Shin sore: bowed swelling on the front of the shin

---

► May or may not be lame – lameness may be evident when horse turns – heat and pain over heels of foot – usually occurs in forefeet – may be visible bulging of coronary band over the quarters of hoof.

Possible diagnosis: Sidebone – *see page 279*

---

► May occur anywhere along length of splint bone – commonly at its junction with cannon bone – heat, pain,

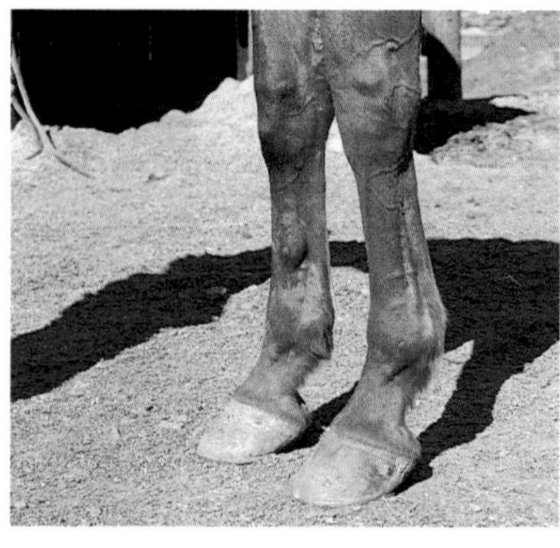

Splint: lump at junction of splint and cannon bones

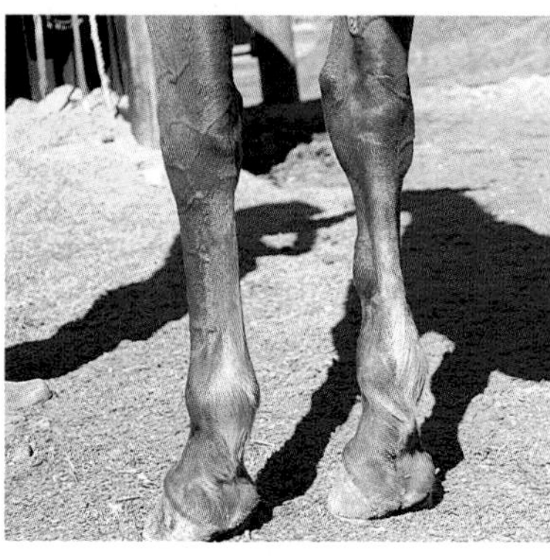

Splint on inside aspect of limb

swelling in affected area – sometimes lameness – as original inflammation subsides enlargement usually becomes smaller but firmer.

Possible diagnosis: Splints – *see page 281*

---

► If enough pressure applied to back of any horse it will flinch and tend to squat – some horses will flinch and squat sometimes to point of sitting like a dog, when only light pressure from tip of a pen is run down either side of spine – when saddled up for riding some horses will straighten back and half squat or arch back as if they are going to buck.

Twitching of tail, restlessness, laying back ears, and inability to stand still indicate back pain.

Some horses, when rider mounts, half squat and often walk off in that position for half a dozen paces before straightening up – during exercise the horse may feel unco-ordinated in hindquarters or may not be able to stretch out properly.

After work when horse hosed down, running water from hose played onto its back may make it squat – when grooming horse, effect of brush on its back may also cause it to squat – keep in mind that some horses with sensitive skin do not like to be groomed.

Possible diagnosis: Spondylitis – *see page 282*

---

► When horse moves or turns, hind limbs are raised alternately with sudden high action as if horse were reacting to sharp pain in foot.

Possible diagnosis: Stringhalt – *see page 284*

---

► Swelling at back of cannon bone between flexor tendons and cannon bone. Horse not usually lame but will not stretch out – pain on palpation of suspensory ligament – may be swelling and pain with pressure where suspensory ligament divides into two branches about 7 cm above fetlock.

Possible diagnosis: Suspensory Ligament Sprain – *see page 286*

---

► Swelling usually involves pastern, fetlock, either side of flexor tendons to just below knee – may be warm to touch but not painful – when pressed with finger temporary depression left in skin – indicates fluid present in tissues underneath – stiffness when moving may be evident.

Possible diagnosis: Swollen Legs – *see page 287*

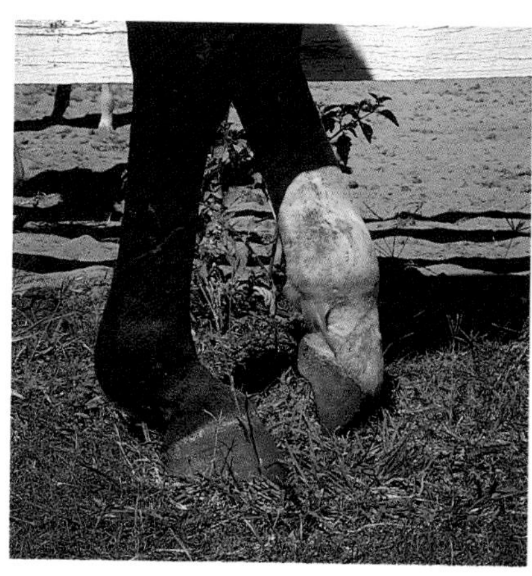

Swollen legs

► Swelling under skin in tendon sheath above point of hock – usually evident on both sides – swelling soft and mobile – more common in young horses – lameness mild and temporary.

Possible diagnosis: Thorough Pin – *see page 289*

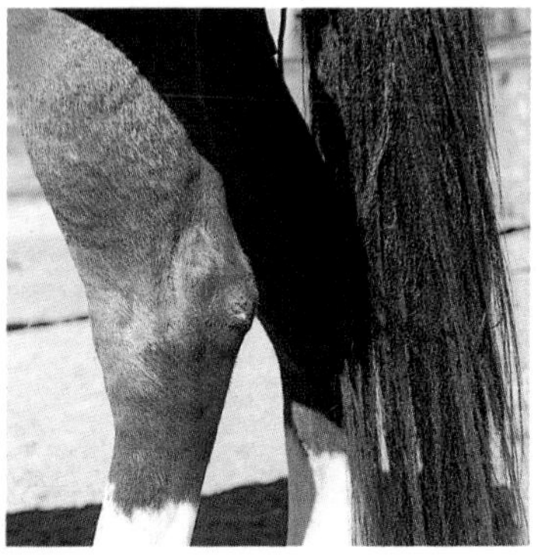

Thorough pin: swelling above the point of the hock

---

► Foul-smelling, black, tarry discharge can be seen in grooves on either side of frog – horse may be lame if sensitive tissues in depths of grooves are involved.

Possible diagnosis: Thrush – *see page 289*

---

► Can vary widely – in mild cases horse steps short in hind limbs, giving the appearance of stiffness during or after exercise – in severe cases horse will show stiffness, pain, sweating and muscle tremor – stiffness involves both hind limbs and forelimbs – may progress to the point where horse cannot move and may lie down. Affected muscles are very hard to touch, indicating cramp – urine may vary in colour from dark brown to reddish black according to severity of the condition.

Possible diagnosis: Tying-Up (Azoturia) – *see page 291*

---

► Horse may be exercised for lengthy periods before lameness evident in hind limbs or severe lameness may be evident immediately after exercise begins – affected hind leg will be cool to touch – shows little or no sign of sweating – rest of body may sweat profusely. Horse shows signs of pain and anxiety – lameness disappears with rest.

Possible diagnosis: Verminous Aneurysm – *see page 294*

---

► Soft, round, fluid-filled swelling – commonly appears on either side of and just above fetlock joint – about 2 cm in diameter.

*Possible diagnosis: Wind Gall – see page 298*

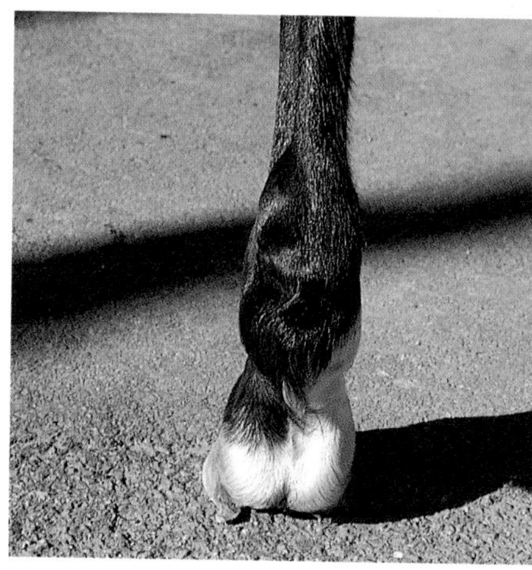

Wind gall on either side and just above the fetlock joint

# LUMPS & SWELLINGS

Find below the group of associated signs that best fits what you observe in your horse.

## ASSOCIATED SIGNS

- Swelling can be seen or felt under skin – when forming in early stages, swelling is diffuse, hot, painful, hard – in later stages is more localised, softer, less painful, forms a point – at this stage when pressed with finger it usually shows a depression – horse may be lethargic, off food, have temperature.

Possible diagnosis: Abscess – *see page 154*

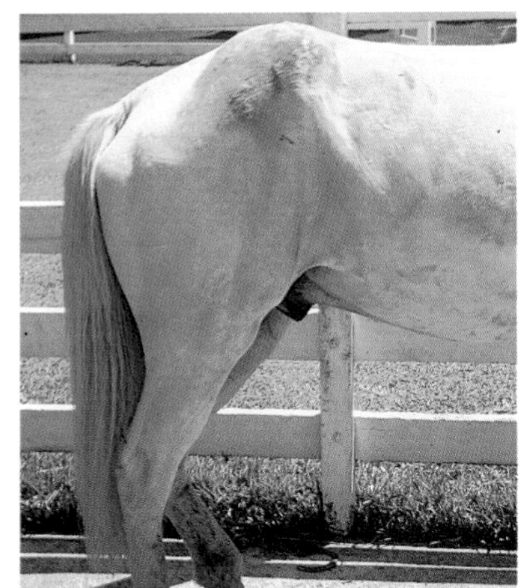

Abscess: hard painful swelling on the rump

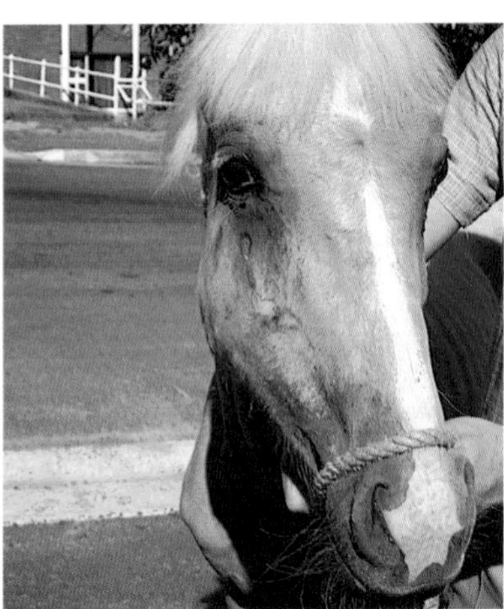

Softer, less painful swelling on the cheek

► Swelling localised in joint(s) – in initial stage (acute) may be firm, warm, swollen, painful to touch – with time (chronic stage) becomes hard – often not warm to touch – less painful – may be restricted movement of joint – eventually permanent joint damage.

Possible diagnosis: Arthritis – *see page 159*

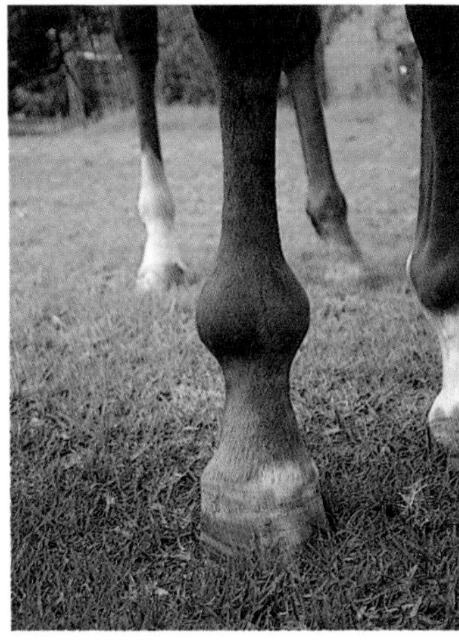

Arthritic fetlock joint

► Shifting lameness – reluctant to move – lying down – swelling around jaw and cheeks in severe cases.

Possible diagnosis: Big Head – *see page 162*

---

► Soft fluid-filled swelling on upper and inner side of hock – more often than not, no heat, pain or lameness.

Possible diagnosis: Bog Spavin – *see page 165*

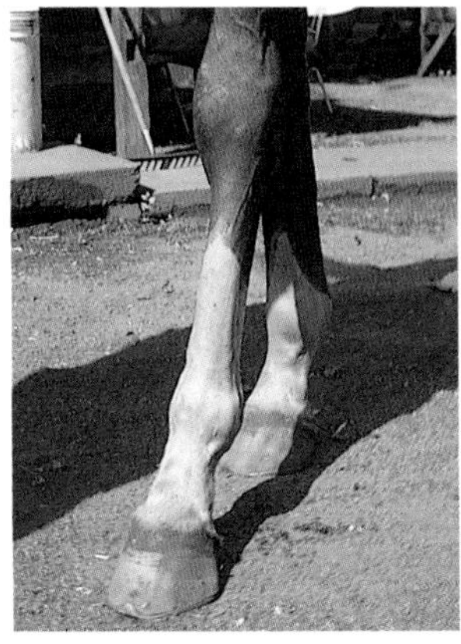

Bog spavin:
soft swelling on the inside of the hock joint

► Hard bony enlargement felt and seen on lower and inner side of hock – horse lame when cold – lameness characterised by reduced flexion of hock and shortening of stride in affected leg – often disappears as horse warms up with exercise – sometimes worsens.

Possible diagnosis: Bone Spavin – *see page 166*

---

► Swelling located in any one of the legs (mainly a front leg) behind cannon bone, running from knee to fetlock. In early stages: swelling – heat – pain on pressure – may step short or be severely lame – in later stages swelling reduced and localised, leaving hard fibrous bow in tendon.

Possible diagnosis: Bowed Tendon – *see page 167*

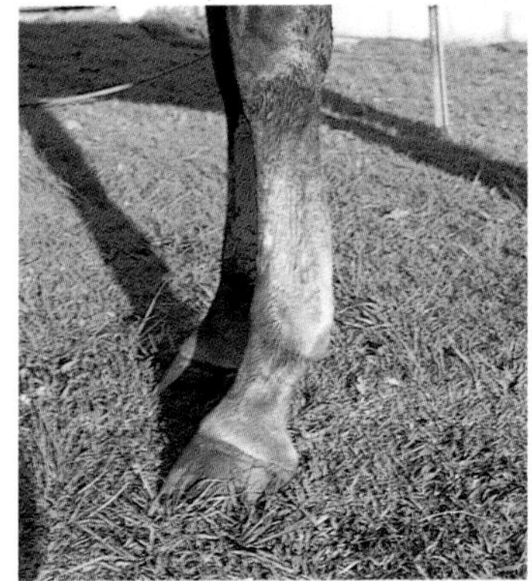

Bow in lower two-thirds of the tendon

► Round, soft, fluid-filled swelling on point of elbow – up to 10 cm in diameter – most cases not sore to touch – lameness slight and temporary.

Possible diagnosis: Capped Elbow (Shoe Boil) – *see page 173*

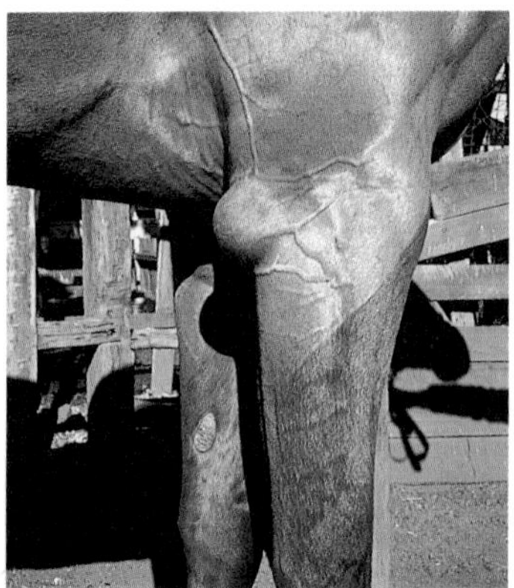

Capped elbow: soft, fluid-filled swelling on the point of the elbow

► Swelling on point of hock – in early stages round, soft, fluid-filled, up to 10 cm in diameter – not sore to touch – lameness, if present, slight and temporary. Old swellings filled with fibrous tissue – hard to touch.

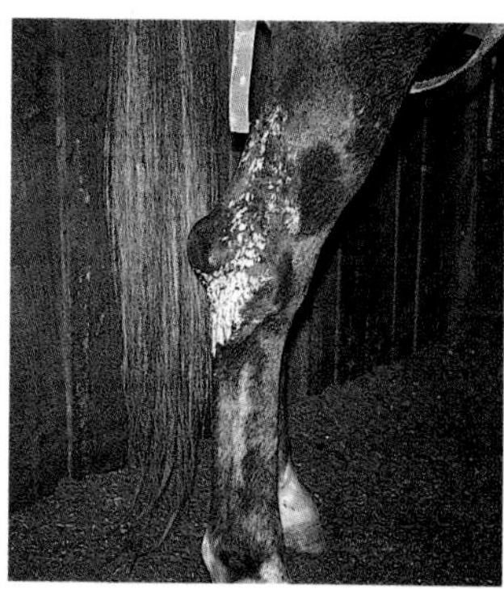

Possible diagnosis:
Capped Hock
– *see page 174*

Capped hock: round swelling on the point of the hock

► Swelling in localised circumscribed area of knee or more generalised – recent swelling soft – older swellings may be very hard – flexibility of knee restricted – signs of pain when knee bent.

Possible diagnosis: Carpitis – *see page 175*

---

► Swelling about 10 cm below point of hock – viewed from side semi-circular in shape – feels hard when pressed.

Possible diagnosis: Curb – *see page 191*

---

► Swelling on one or both sides of withers – hot to touch – painful – may erupt, discharging straw-coloured fluid – in few days discharge changes to whitish-yellow pus.

Possible diagnosis: Fistulous Withers – *see page 203*

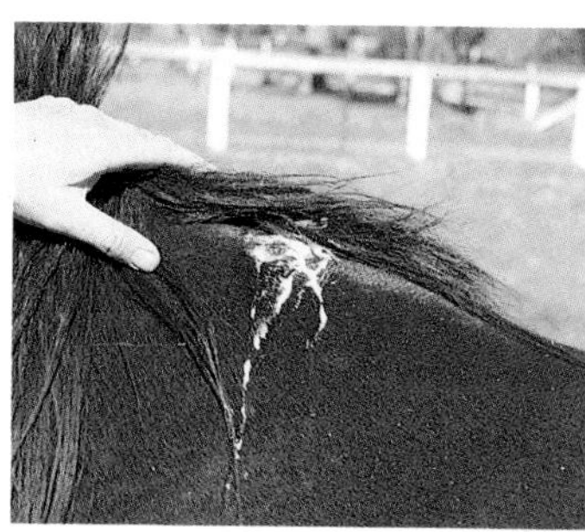

Fistulous withers:
pus discharge is evident

► May be discharge from one or both nostrils depending on whether one or both guttural pouches are involved – often nasal discharge obvious when horse puts head to ground. Swelling below ear, on one or both sides – where head meets neck – discomfort – breathing difficult. When tapped with fingers swelling may be firm, containing pus, or make hollow sound indicating it contains air.

Possible diagnosis: Guttural Pouch, Infected (contains pus) or Guttural Pouch — Tympany (contains trapped air) – *see page 217*

---

► Generally occurs in area of muscle masses – size varies up to that of a football – usually not sore to touch – in early stage soft to touch – when tapped feels like fluid-filled cavity.

Possible diagnosis: Haematoma – *see page 218*

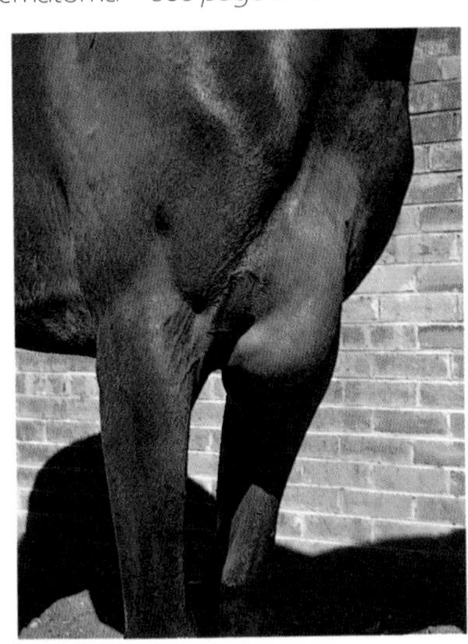

Haematoma: blood-filled swelling

► Heat, pain and swelling in affected joint(s) of new-born foal – lameness – stiffness in movement – temperature rise.

Possible diagnosis: Joint ill – *see page 229*

---

► Swollen membrane of hard palate – if extends below level of tables of incisor teeth may cause discomfort when eating – horse may go off feed.

Possible diagnosis: Lampas – *see page 236*

► Udder may be larger on one side – painful to touch, hot, swollen, hard, sometimes lumpy – milk may be thick and discoloured – may have temperature.

Possible diagnosis: Mastitis – *see page 239*

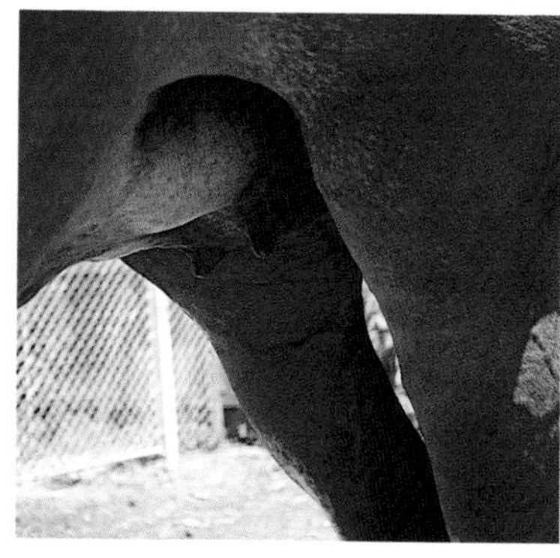

Mastitis: swollen udder

► Small (1 cm) to large (10 cm) dark lumps – usually located around anus or vulva, under tail, occasionally on or near eyelids – found frequently on old grey horses.

Possible diagnosis: Melanoma – *see page 239*

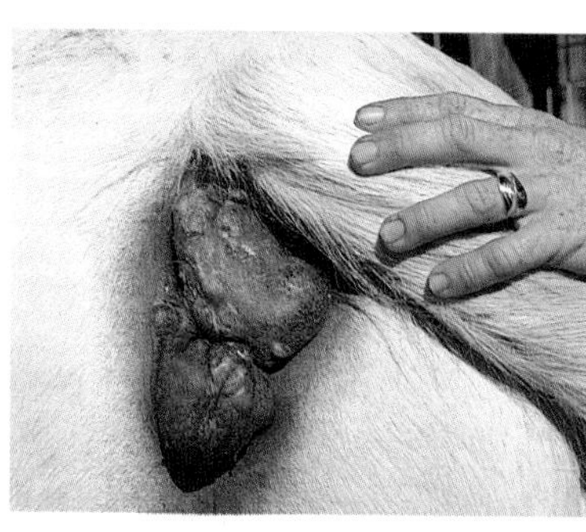

Melanoma under the tail

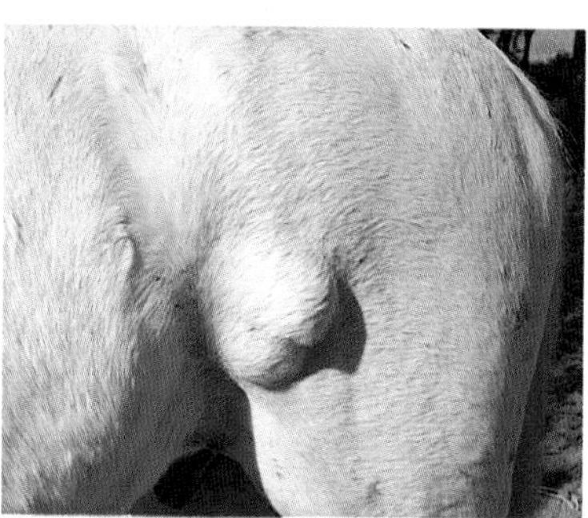

Melanoma: a large swelling on the upper thigh

► Swelling appears just above or below front of fetlock – usually hard – pain on bending fetlock and lameness are present.

Possible diagnosis: Osselets – *see page 245*

---

► Tenderness around poll – painful, well-defined, or diffuse, ill-defined, swelling may be seen – stiffness in head movement – pus discharge in mane – may be noticed when putting on bridle.

Possible diagnosis: Poll Evil – *see page 263*

---

► Swelling on front or sides of pastern – in early stages evidence of heat, swelling, pain on pressure, lameness – in later stages bony swelling varying in size can be seen and felt on pastern.

Possible diagnosis: Ringbone – *see page 270*

---

► Skin tumour located mainly on head, shoulders, lower limbs – appears as one or several wart-like lumps – size varies 1–10 cm in diameter – may have thick crusty surface or ulcerated, raw, fleshy one that bleeds readily when touched.

Possible diagnosis: Sarcoid – *see page 274*

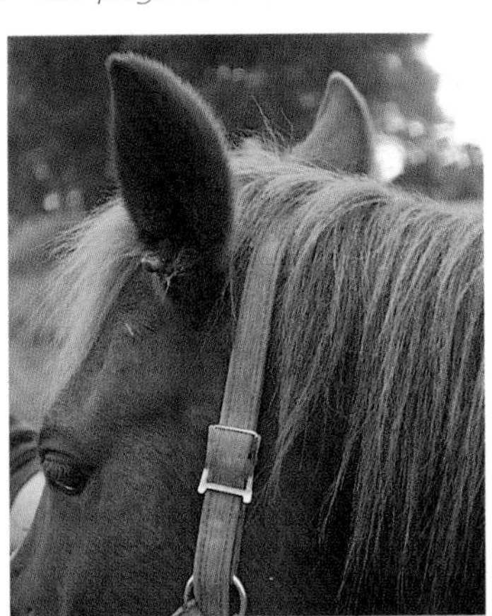

Sarcoid: lump at the base of the ear

► Swelling at back of fetlock – lameness – pain on application of pressure to sesamoid bones and on bending fetlock joint.

Possible diagnosis: Sesamoiditis – *see page 277*

► Swelling on front of cannon bone – one or both forelimbs involved – warm and painful to touch – horse may show lameness or shortening of stride.

Possible diagnosis: Shin Soreness – *see page 278*

---

► May occur anywhere along length of splint bone – commonly at its junction with cannon bone – heat, pain, swelling in affected area – sometimes lameness – as original inflammation subsides, enlargement usually becomes smaller but firmer.

Possible diagnosis: Splints – *see page 281*

---

► Lymph nodes of head and neck swollen – those under jaw most noticeable – loss of appetite – thick discharge from both nostrils – cough – temperature.

Possible diagnosis: Strangles – *see page 283*

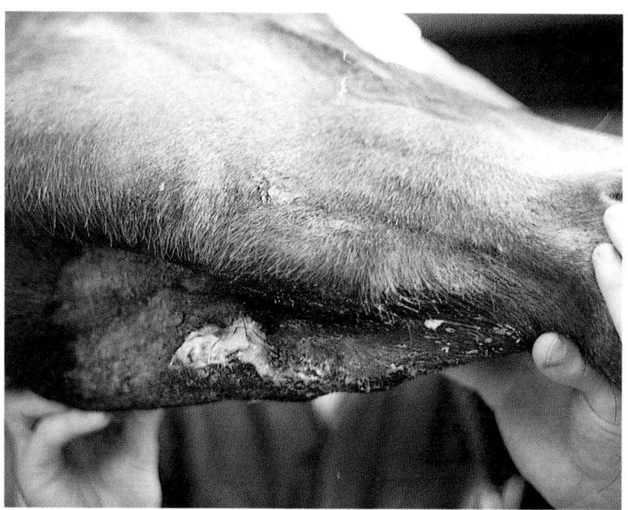

Strangles: discharge from a lump beneath the skin can be seen under the jaw

► Swelling usually involves pastern, fetlock, either side of flexor tendons to just below knee – may be warm to touch but not painful – when pressed with finger temporary depression left in skin – indicates fluid present in tissues underneath – stiffness when moving may be evident.

Possible diagnosis: Swollen Legs – *see page 287*

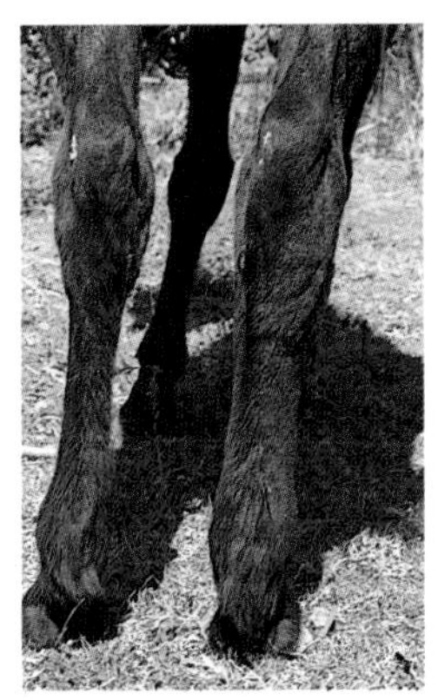

Swollen leg: swelling either side of flexor tendons

► Swelling under skin in tendon sheath above point of hock – usually evident on both sides – swelling soft and mobile – more common in young horses.

Possible diagnosis: Thorough Pin – *see page 289*

---

► Swelling located on one or both sides of upper section of windpipe – firm, mobile, oval-shaped, 4–7 cm across.

Possible diagnosis: Thyroid Gland Enlargement – *see page 290*

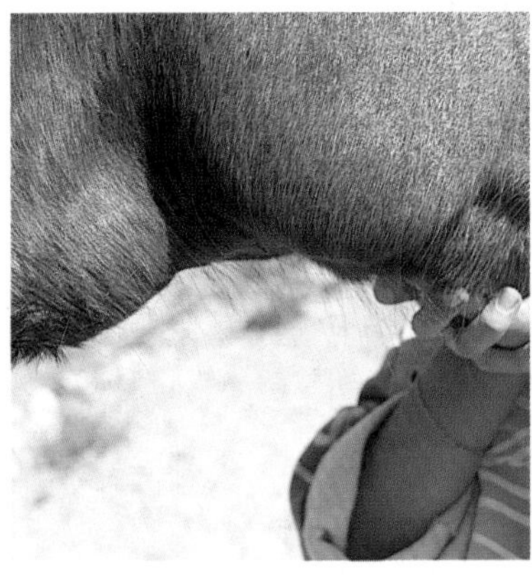

Enlarged thyroid gland

► Round, hard, immobile swelling 4–14 cm across on outside of hind leg below stifle – usually first noticed in weanlings and yearlings – as a rule no lameness.

Possible diagnosis: Tumoral Calcinosis (Calcified Swelling) – *see page 291*

► Swelling in region of navel – may be up to 5 cm in diameter.

Possible diagnosis: Umbilical Hernia – *see page 293*

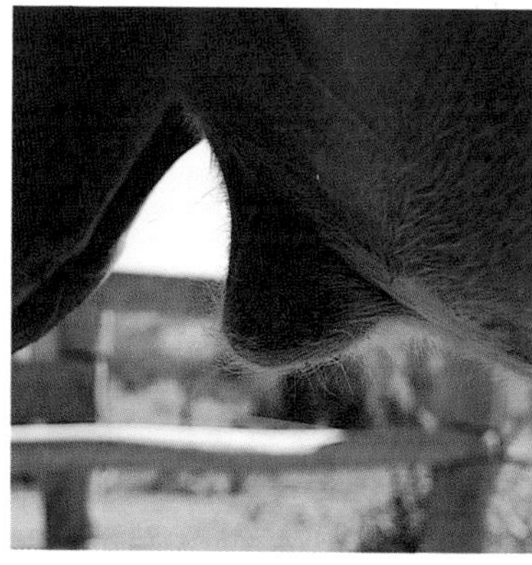

Umbilical hernia

► Lumps varying in size from 2 mm to 2 cm – common sites are nose, lips, eyelids and cheeks – colour from pink to grey – have raised, rough, horny surfaces.

Possible diagnosis: Warts – *see page 296*

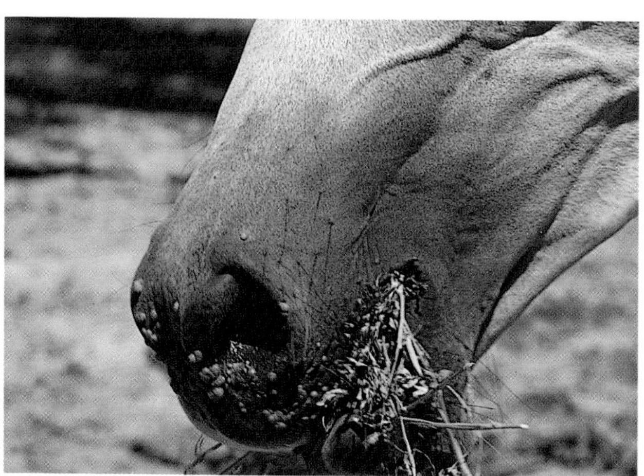

Warts around the nose

► Soft, round, fluid-filled swelling – commonly appears on either side of and just above fetlock joint – about 2 cm in diameter.

Possible diagnosis: Wind Gall – *see page 298*

# NASAL DISCHARGE

Find below the group of associated signs that best fits what you observe in your horse.

## ASSOCIATED SIGNS

► Obvious sign is horse bleeding from one or both nostrils after race, track work or sometimes swimming – bleeding may begin during exercise, immediately after, or sometimes hours after exercise has finished – blood may lie inside nostrils, drip to ground, or flow freely. Some horses bleed in the lungs – only signs of this may be laboured breathing, distress and coughing – often the more serious type of haemorrhage.

Possible diagnosis:
Bleeder (Epistaxis)
– *see page 164*

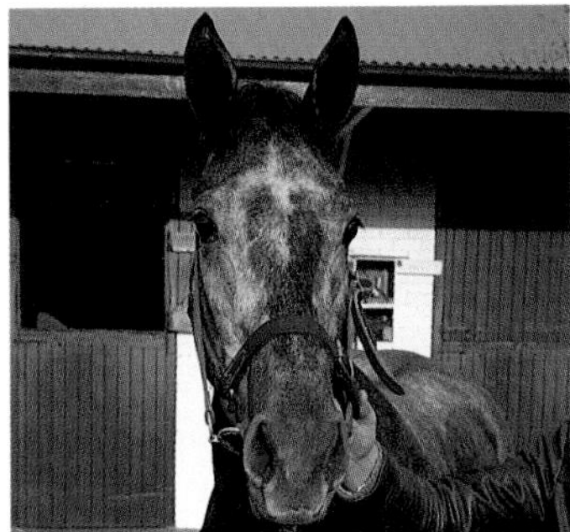

Blood trickling from both nostrils

► Clear watery discharge from both nostrils – persistent hacking cough – clear watery discharge from eyes – may be normal between bouts of coughing attacks.

Possible diagnosis: Bronchial Asthma (Allergic Bronchitis) – *see page 170*

---

► Dry cough – discharge from both nostrils, initially clear and watery, progressing to thick mucus – temperature – loss of appetite – lethargy.

Possible diagnosis:
Equine Influenza
– *see page 201*

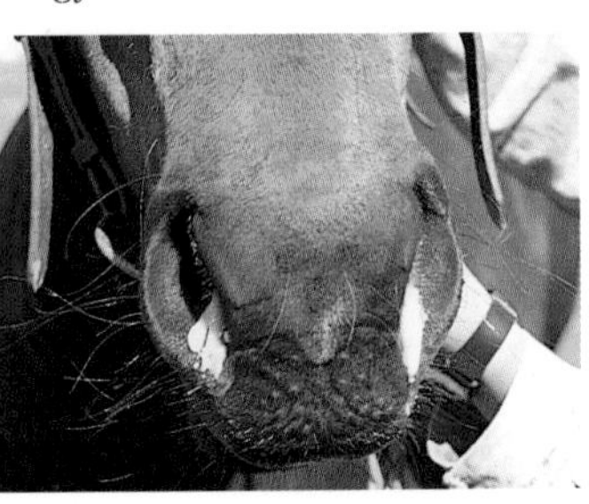

Creamy, purulent discharge from both nostrils

► Pregnant mares may abort during illness or shortly after — incubation period of 2–6 days – symptoms may be high temperature (42°C) – off food – dopey – weak – inflamed, discoloured eyes. Some show oedema (swelling) in legs, underbelly and udder – constipation – colic – diarrhoea.

Possible diagnosis: Equine Viral Arteritis – *see page 202*

---

► Incubation period of infection about 2 weeks – symptoms of a cold – temperature up – coughing – sneezing – respiratory disease – abortion may occur up to 4 months after infection when mare appears healthy – abortion usually occurs from 5th month onwards. Foetus expelled rapidly with placenta – virus can affect brain and spinal cord of mare causing paralysis of hindquarters – foetus aborted after 6 months shows discolouration of placental fluid and hooves due to diarrhoea in uterus. Disease found throughout world including Australia.

Possible diagnosis: Equine Viral Rhinopneumonitis – *see page 202*

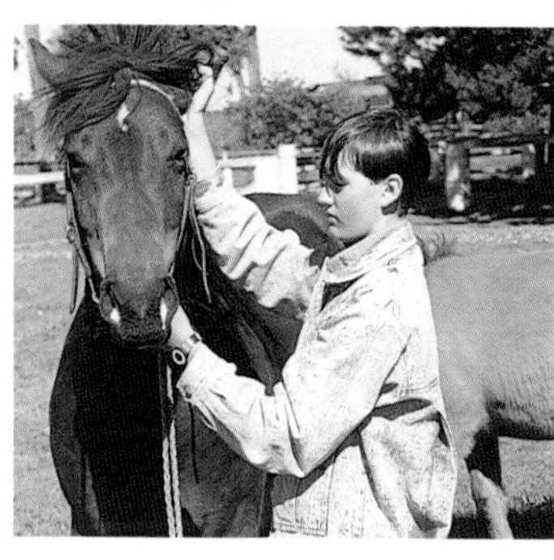

Pus discharge from nostrils

► Young foals with purulent discharge from both nostrils – rattling sound in chest – coughing – laboured breathing – often stimulated by handling – harsh coat – elevated temperature.

Possible diagnosis: Foal Pneumonia (Rattles) – *see page 204*

---

► Weight loss – coughing – rapid shallow respiration – hear moisture in chest – ulcerations of nasal cavity and skin – often erupting on inside of hock – nodules under skin are up to 2 cm in diameter and discharge a honey-like pus.

Possible diagnosis: Glanders – *see page 216*

- Discharge from one or both nostrils depending on whether one or both guttural pouches are involved – often nasal discharge obvious when horse puts head to ground. Swelling below ear, on one or both sides – where head meets neck – discomfort – breathing difficult. When tapped with fingers, swelling may be firm, containing pus (infected), or make hollow sound indicating it contains air (tympany).

Possible diagnosis: Guttural Pouch, Infected or Guttural Pouch – Tympany – *see page 217*

---

- Discharge from both nostrils – off food – lethargic – rapid shallow respiration – cough – high temperature – breath may have foul odour – hear moisture in chest as horse breathes in and out – doesn't want to move or lie down – nostrils may be flared.

Possible diagnosis: Pneumonia – *see page 261*

---

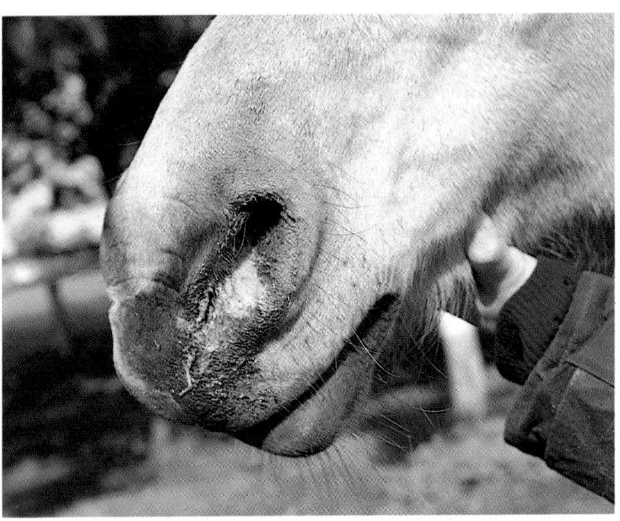

Sinusitis: pus discharge from one nostril

- Discharge from one nostril, thick and foul-smelling, possibly streaked with blood – may be swelling above or below eye – may be discharge from eye – if sinus full of pus it emits dull sound when tapped.

Possible diagnosis: Sinusitis – *see page 279*

---

► Copious, purulent discharge from both nostrils – loss of appetite – slight cough – lymph nodes under jaw inflamed and swollen – temperature – laboured respiration.

Possible diagnosis: Strangles – *see page 283*

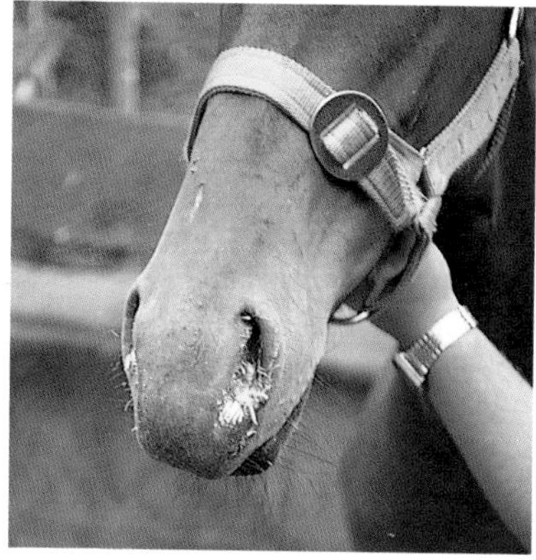

Strangles: both nostrils discharging

---

► Clear or purulent mucus sometimes tinged with blood – from one nostril – abnormal sound coming from nostril especially when horse worked – may be no movement of air in or out of nostril – detected by placing hand over nostril – may be swelling of one side of nasal cavity in association with watery and bulging eye.

Possible diagnosis: Tumour – *see page 291*

# NERVOUS SYSTEM DISORDERS

Find below the group of associated signs that best fits what you observe in your horse.

## BACKGROUND

Call your veterinarian if your horse shows signs of excitement, over-reaction to normal external stimuli, depression, staggering, knuckling over, walking in circles, collapse, general muscle tremor, rigidity, paddling movements of legs, paralysis, blindness and/or coma.

While waiting for the veterinarian, place the horse in an area where it will cause minimal damage to itself. Provide fluids and protection from environment (warmth or shade), and reduce external stimuli to a minimum by keeping the noise level down and handling the horse as little as possible.

Causes are numerous:

1. Viruses e.g. eastern equine encephalomyelitis (EEE), western equine encephalomyelitis (WEE)

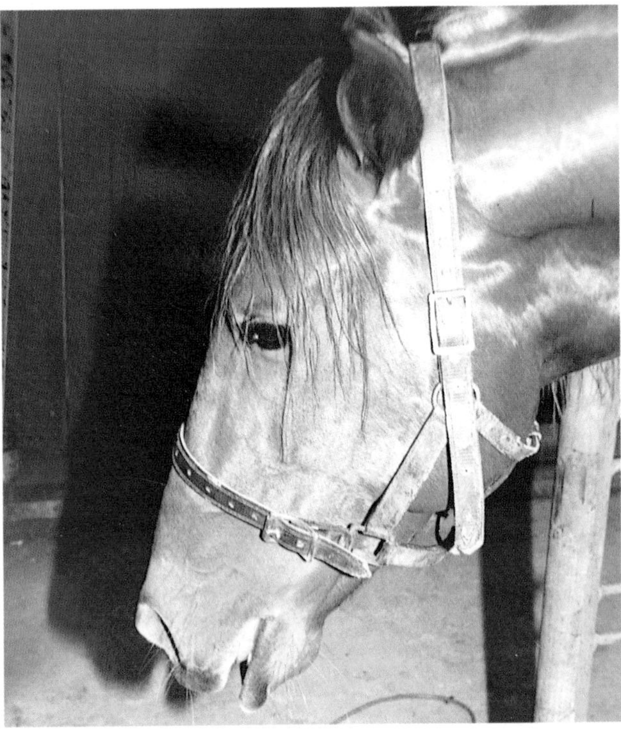

This horse is depressed

and Venezuelan equine encephalomyelitis (VEE) – all limited to America;
2. Bacteria e.g. tetanus;
3. Trauma e.g. injury;
4. Tumours;
5. Poisonous plants e.g. *Indigophera dominii* causes Birdsville disease and *Atalaya hemiglauca* causes Kimberley or Walkabout disease in Australia;
6. Poisonous chemicals.

The signs are visible expressions of encephalitis (inflammation of the brain) or meningitis (inflammation of the meninges i.e. the membranes covering the surface of the brain).

## ASSOCIATED SIGNS

► Found in Germany – more common among horses 3–6 years of age – lethargy – chewing slowly, eventually unable to chew or swallow – compulsive circling – skin becomes hypersensitive. Signs worsen progressively over 1–3 weeks leading to death in 70–90% of cases.

Possible diagnosis: Borna Disease – *see page 166*

---

► Difficulty in grasping food with lips and teeth – drools saliva – unable to drink – paralysis of tongue – slow mastication – unable to swallow – wobbliness in fore and hindquarters – knuckling over – stumbling – collapse with constant paddling movements of limbs leading to death.

Possible diagnosis: Botulism – *see page 167*

---

► Yawning – sleepiness – depraved appetite – irritability – unco-ordinated – twitching of head and neck muscles – walking in a straight line – may stand for hours pushing against immovable objects – reluctant to lie down – urine red to brown colour – mucous membranes may be jaundiced – over period of weeks extreme weight loss – eventually unable to get up – coma – death. Occurs in Western Australia and Northern Territory.

Possible diagnosis: Kimberley (Walkabout) Disease – *see page 230*

---

► Found in Europe and US – early signs: drools saliva – spastic lip movement – hyperexcitable – leading to depression and not eating. Rare cases become aggressive (biting and kicking). Paralysis develops – first affecting the ability to swallow and vocal cords (altered whinny) – then spreads to hindquarters with collapse and death in 2–7 days after initial signs.

Possible diagnosis: Rabies – *see page 268*

---

► Stiffness – rigidity of whole body – third eyelids partially cover the eyes – difficulty with taking food into mouth and chewing – drooling a mixture of saliva and food – general stiffness leads to convulsions and death in up to 80% of cases.

Possible diagnosis: Tetanus – *see page 288*

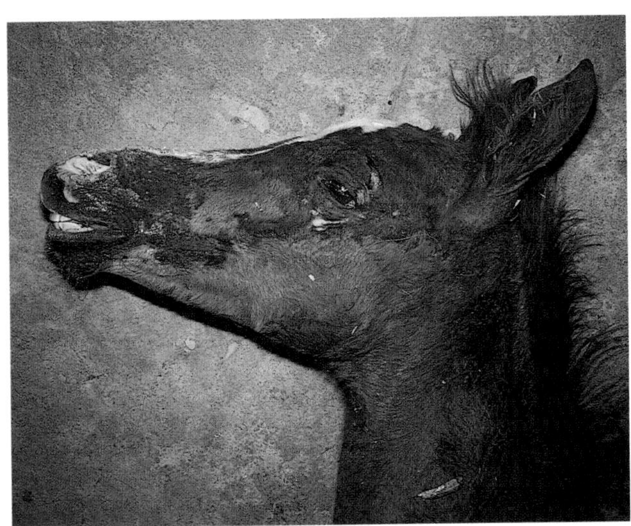

Tetanus (lockjaw): muscle spasms of the head

---

► Poor co-ordination – wobbling – weakness – clumsiness – not wanting to lie down or roll. Condition may remain static or progress from slight wobbling to exaggerated, drunken movements, with horse crashing into objects and obstacles such as doorways. Generally recognised in horses 1–2 years of age when being broken in, educated and exercised.

Possible diagnosis: Wobbler – *see page 298*

# PALE GUMS & CONJUNCTIVA

Find below the group of associated signs that best fits what you observe in your horse.

## BACKGROUND

Pale mucous membranes (gums and conjunctiva) are a sign of anaemia. Anaemia is not a disease, it is a symptom of something else, so it is essential to find the causal factor(s) before treatment is initiated. Anaemia is a decrease in haemoglobin and/or red blood cells to level(s) below normal, thus reducing the oxygen-carrying capacity of the blood. A stressed horse, e.g. one in hard training and performing frequently, will readily show signs of anaemia. On the other hand, an unstressed horse which is anaemic may not show any other signs at all.

## ASSOCIATED SIGNS

► Bleeding – external or internal – due to some form of injury. Pale conjunctiva and gums – weakness.

Possible diagnosis: Anaemia, due to bleeding — *see page 155*

---

► Temperature of horse high, maybe up to 41.5°C – dull – unsteady – swelling of limbs and trunk – blood in urine – anaemic – presence of ticks – occurs mostly in tropics and sub-tropics where conditions suitable for survival of tick – may be fatal.

Possible diagnosis: Babesiosis (Piroplasmosis) – *see page 162*

---

► Temperature – pale gums and conjunctiva (inside eyelids), sometimes yellow with jaundice – not eating –

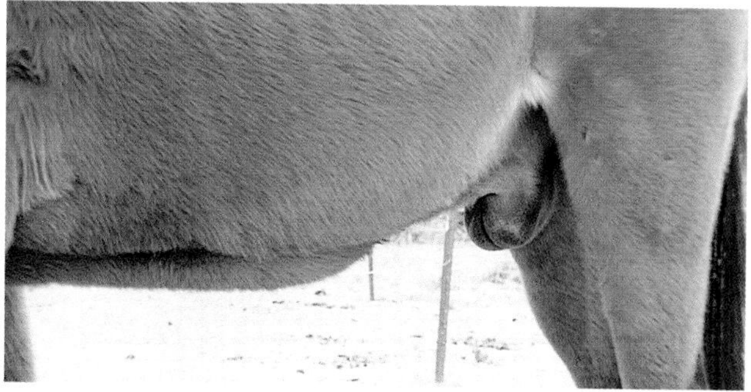

Fluid swelling under the belly

weight loss – weakness – fluid swelling under belly and in legs – clear discharge from eyes and nose.

Possible diagnosis: Equine Infectious Anaemia – *see page 200*

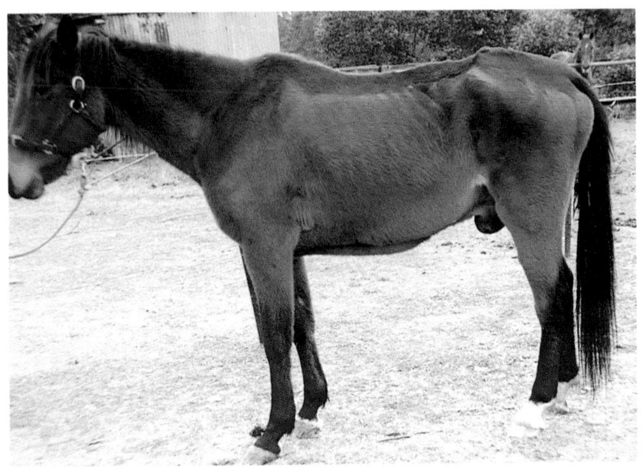

Signs of weight loss

---

► Found in new-born foal – sluggish – dull – weak – no longer suckles – lies down – rapid shallow breathing (panting), especially after exercise – anaemic (pale gums and conjunctiva) – then gums and conjunctiva change to varying shades of yellow – after 24 hours urine dark brown in colour – may collapse.

Possible diagnosis: Isoimmune Haemolytic Jaundice – *see page 228*

---

► Pale mucous membranes – dull harsh coat – weight loss – poor performance – poor appetite.

Possible diagnosis: Nutritional Deficiency Anaemia – *see page 156*

---

► Weight loss – dull harsh coat – pot belly – pale mucous membranes of eyelids and gums – diarrhoea – tail rubbing – poor appetite – reduced performance – poor

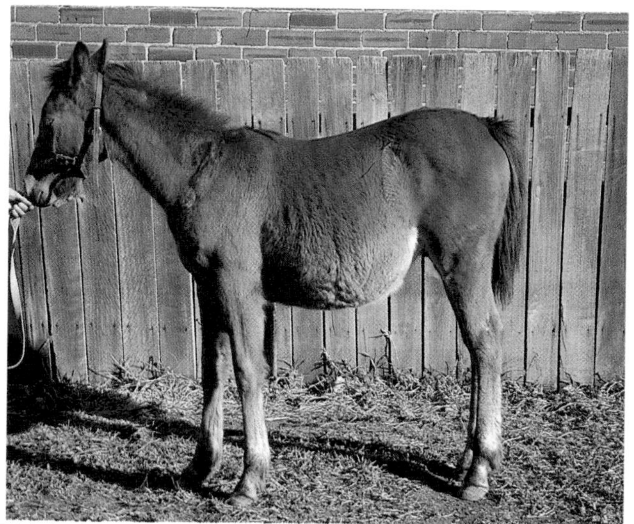

This foal shows typical signs of worms: a dull harsh coat, weight loss and a pot belly

stamina – colic – coughing in young foals – botfly eggs on coat.

Possible diagnosis: Parasites (worms) – *see page 248*

# POOR PERFORMANCE

Find below the group of associated signs that best fits what you observe in your horse.

## BACKGROUND

This section is not concerned with horses that don't perform well because they lack ability, are poorly trained or incorrectly raced. It deals only with horses that have ability but because of disease or injury do not achieve maximum fitness and fail to perform to the best of their ability.

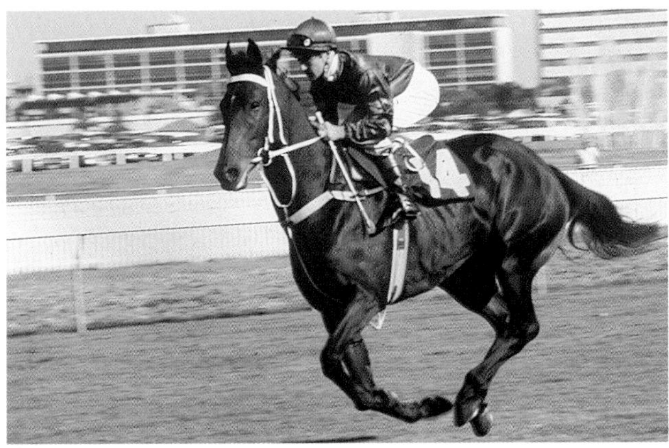

Horse galloping at the peak of its performance

## ASSOCIATED SIGNS

► Lethargy – loss of appetite – restlessness – loss of condition – poor coat – poor performance. Colour of tissue around eye (conjunctiva) and gums reflects status of red blood cells in horse – normal colour is pink – white indicates severe anaemia – in many cases the colour does not fall into either category.

Possible diagnosis: Anaemia – *see pages 155–8*

---

► Dry harsh coat – sunken eyes – lethargy – loss of appetite – hard, dry ball of manure – fatigue – cramping – tying up – lack of will to win – poor recovery from exercise – when skin pinched, lack of return or slow return to normal.

Possible diagnosis: Dehydration – *see page 193*

---

► Poor exercise tolerance and fatigue – laboured, rapid breathing and rapid heart rate following moderate exercise – respiration and heart rate take a long time to return to normal after exercise.

Possible diagnosis: Heart Disease – *see page 219*

---

► Appears in horses 5 years or older – signs appear gradually – most prominent sign is exaggerated and lengthy expiration (breathing out) especially during or after exercise – over period of time breathing difficult, even at rest – horse develops barrel chest to help compensate – wheezing associated with short, shallow cough evident.

Possible diagnosis: Heaves (Broken Wind) – *see page 222*

---

► Signs may vary markedly – horse may not be stretching out – stepping short – favouring a leg – nodding head – stilted, proppy action – changing leading leg – rough action.

Possible diagnosis: Lameness – *see page 86*

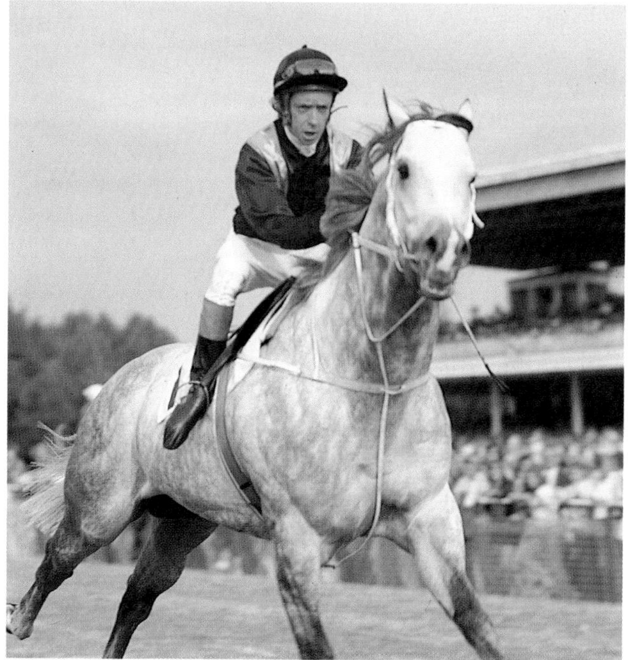

Good performance — this horse is fully stretched

- A peculiar noise, ranging from a whistle to a roar, that some horses make when they breathe in (inspiration) – most horses only show signs of the noise when galloping fully extended – a minority show signs even at rest. Horse's ability to perform in events where there is stress on respiratory system is adversely affected – most often occurs in horses 16 hands or more in height and aged 3–7 years – rare in ponies.

Possible diagnosis: Roaring – *see page 272*

---

- Noise during strenuous exercise, e.g. extended gallop – often towards end of race – horse makes a choking noise – may be associated with breathing in and out.

Possible diagnosis: Soft Palate Displacement – *see page 280*

---

- During or after work horse steps short in hind limbs, giving appearance of stiffness – only sign may be that horse will not stretch out during training or when competing – horses with these signs normally on high-grain diet and only show signs when worked after a day or more of rest.

Possible diagnosis: Tying-Up – *see page 291*

---

- Lack of muscle – thinness – poor appetite – bony prominences more pronounced – obvious loss of weight.

Possible diagnosis: Weight Loss – *see page 297*

# SKIN CONDITION

Find below the group of associated signs that best fits what you observe in your horse.

## ASSOCIATED SIGNS

► Inability to sweat – observed in horses in tropical countries – more commonly among horses imported from temperate zones – within few weeks horse sweats less – sweating may be confined to localised areas such as crest of neck, under chest – skin dry, inelastic and flaky – very high temperatures after exercise (43°C) – severe respiratory distress – may affect horse born in tropics.

Possible diagnosis: Anhydrosis (Inability to Sweat; Dry Coat) – *see page 158*

---

► Swelling with or without ulceration – common sites are third eyelid (nictitating membrane), eyelids and penis.

Possible diagnosis: Cancer (Squamous Cell Carcinoma) – *see page 173*

---

► Numerous small nodules with minute scab on top – found on neck, cheeks, rump, lower limbs – small lumps are itchy, often with hair standing up – usually appear during summer months.

Possible diagnosis: Fly and Mosquito Bites – *see page 204*

---

► Inflammation of skin at back of pastern between heels – more frequently in hind limbs than forelimbs – in early stages sore to touch, raw and bleeds – hair loss and deep cracks develop with thickened skin – swelling of pastern and fetlock may accompany lameness.

Possible diagnosis: Greasy Heel – *see page 216*

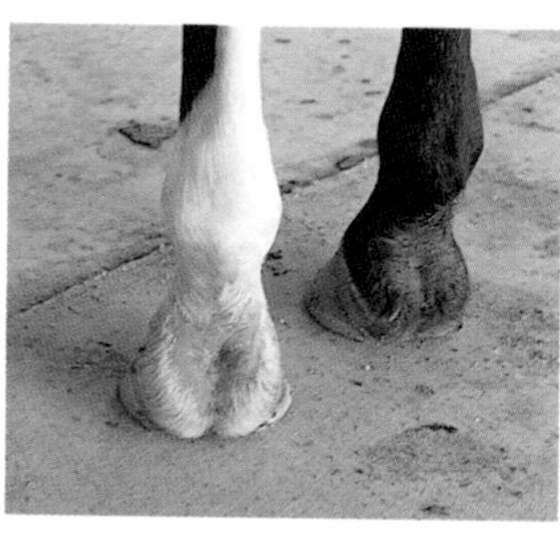

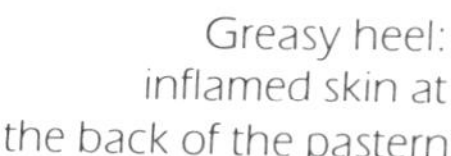

Greasy heel: inflamed skin at the back of the pastern

► Severe irritation – mainly confined to legs below knees and hocks – may involve armpits, inner thighs, belly. Muzzle and nose may become involved by horse rubbing legs with its muzzle. Skin in affected areas is red – oozes serum which forms into hard crusts – in chronic cases skin forms thickened folds. Hair on legs broken from constant rubbing – assumes moth-eaten appearance.

Possible diagnosis: Leg Mange – *see page 236*

---

► Severe irritation of skin – rubbing, biting, scratching, coat dull – some hair falls out – horse assumes motley appearance – long hair of mane and tail matted – loss of condition. If hair parted lice can be seen under good light.

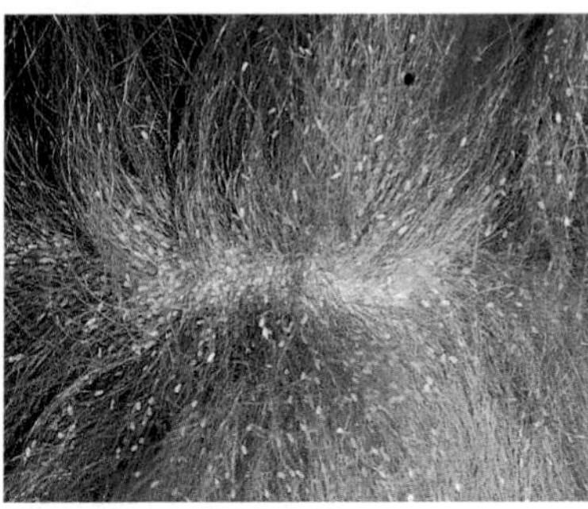

Possible diagnosis: Lice – *see page 237*

Sucking lice in the long hair

---

► Small (1 cm) to large (10 cm or more) dark lumps – may be located around anus or vulva – under tail – occasionally on or near eyelids – more frequently seen in old grey horses.

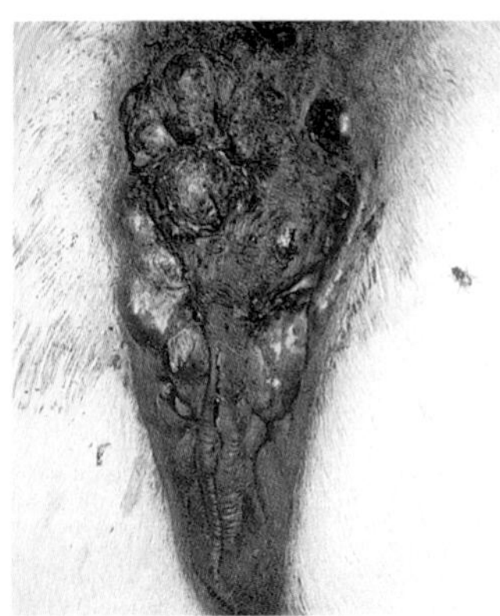

Possible diagnosis: Melanoma – *see page 239*

Melanoma around the anus

► Circular areas of hair loss – 2 cm in diameter – around head, neck and ventral abdomen – scaly appearance of skin – itchiness – looks similar to ringworm.

Possible diagnosis: Onchocerciasis – *see page 243*

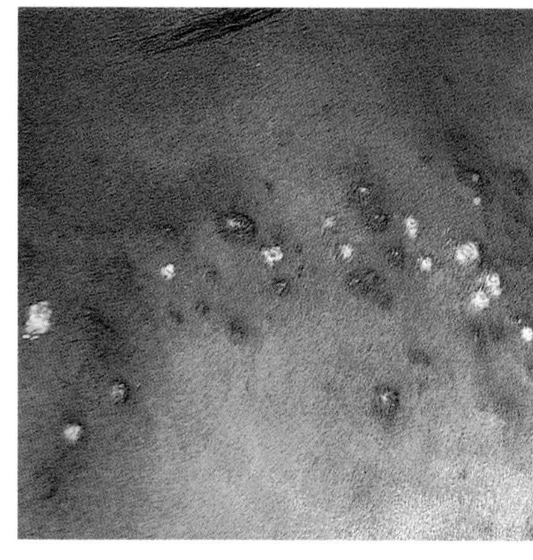

Onchocerciasis: circular areas of hair loss

---

► Itching, rubbing, biting – hair loss – abrasion of skin – mainly in areas of ears, mane, withers and tail – in longstanding cases skin becomes thickened, wrinkled and discoloured, with sparse hair cover.

Possible diagnosis: Queensland Itch – *see page 266*

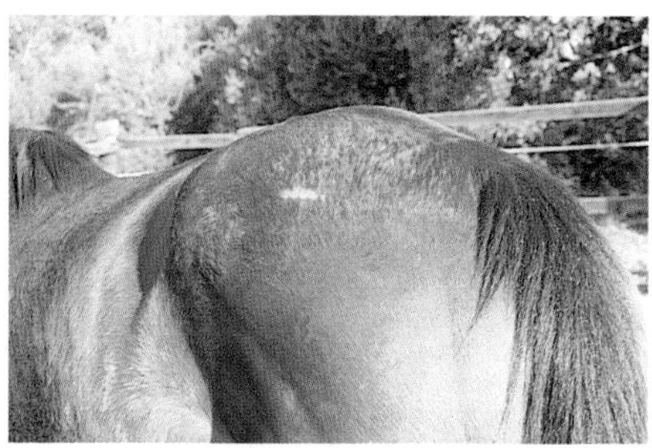

Queensland itch on the rump

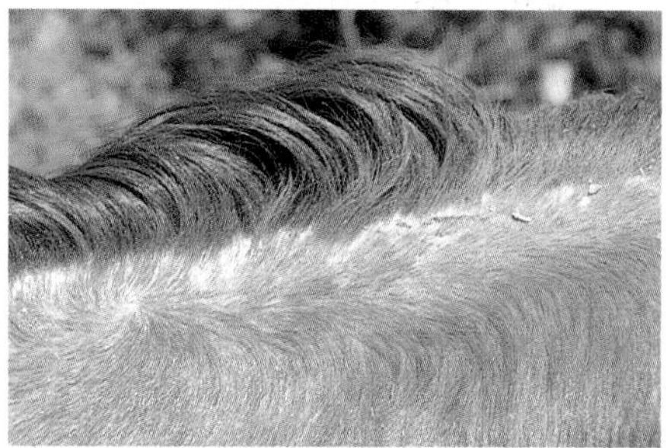

Queensland itch in the mane

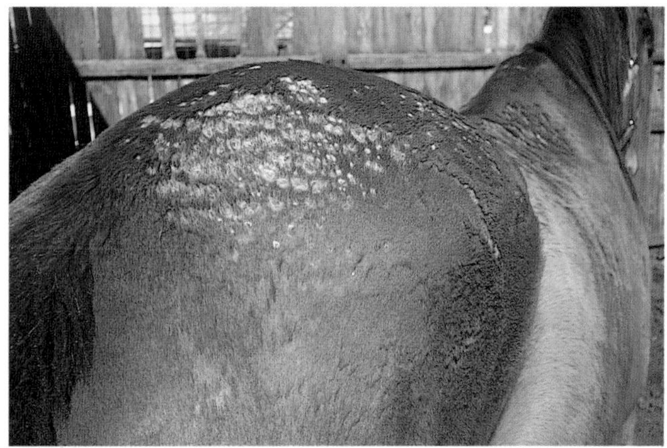

Rain scald on the rump

► Hair on back and croup matted with inflammatory fluid that oozes from skin – some clumps of matted hair fall out – others, if peeled off, leave raw bleeding surface.

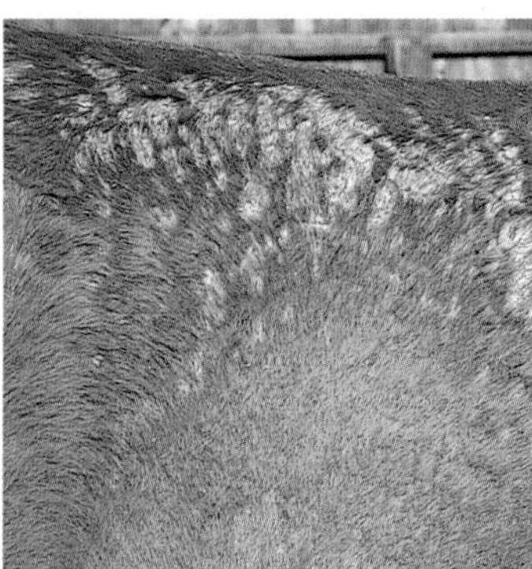

Possible diagnosis:
Rain Scald
– *see page 268*

Rain scald along the back

---

► Circular area of raised hair 1–3 cm in diameter – hair becomes brittle – falls out about 10 days after infection – circular clumps can be plucked out – leave moist,

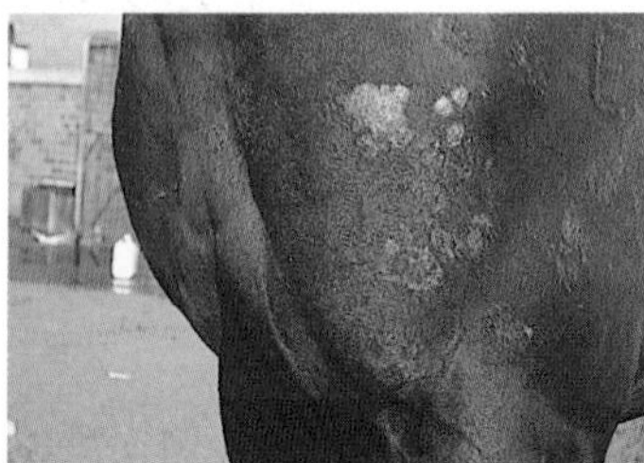

Ringworm: hair loss on the shoulder

circular, hairless lesions – sometimes dotted with few spots of blood – mainly found on head, girth and shoulders – may have wider distribution.

Possible diagnosis: Ringworm – *see page 271*

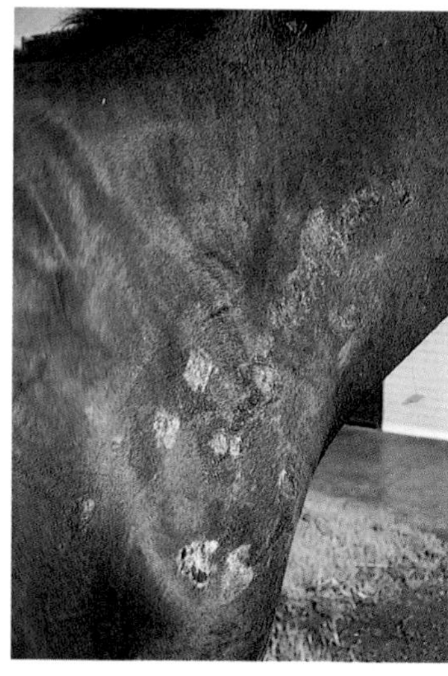

Ringworm: extensive hair loss on shoulders and neck

---

► Hair is rubbed off and skin broken on side of wither or under girth – result of constant pressure or rubbing – often leaves raw, bleeding sores – vary in size – slow to heal.

Possible diagnosis: Saddle Sore; Girth Gall – *see page 274*

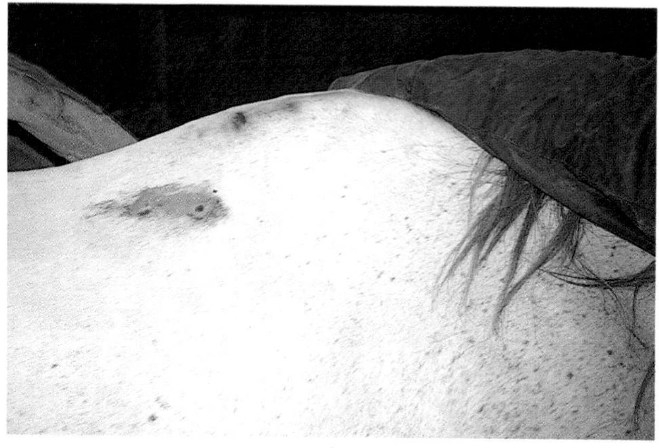

Saddle sore

► Usually located on head, shoulders or lower limbs – one or several wart-like growths – vary in size from 1–10 cm in diameter – thick crusty surface – or may be raw, ulcerated, fleshy surface that bleeds freely when touched.

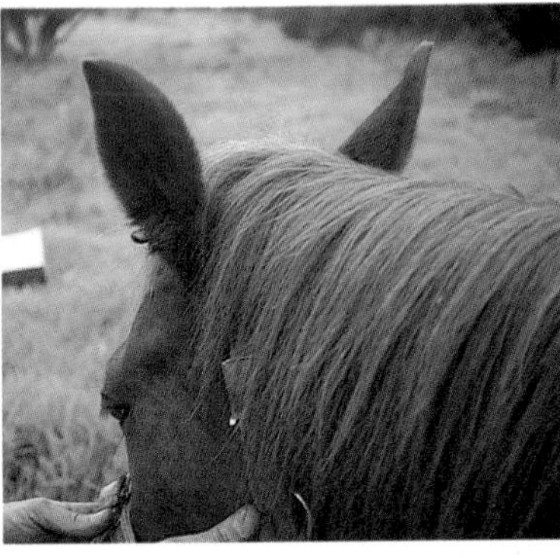

Possible diagnosis: Sarcoid – *see page 274*

Sarcoid at the base of the ear

---

► Severe irritation – initially on head and neck – extending to other parts of body – does not involve mane, tail or lower limbs – small nodules form – often with a scab on top – hair loss – moth-eaten appearance – skin becomes thickened – forms into folds – weight loss.

Itchy red spots form on inside of forearms and exposed skin of stablehands having close contact with horse.

Possible diagnosis: Sarcoptic Mange (Scabies) – *see page 276*

---

► Fleshy tissue develops from wound or moist skin in region of eye, penis or prepuce.

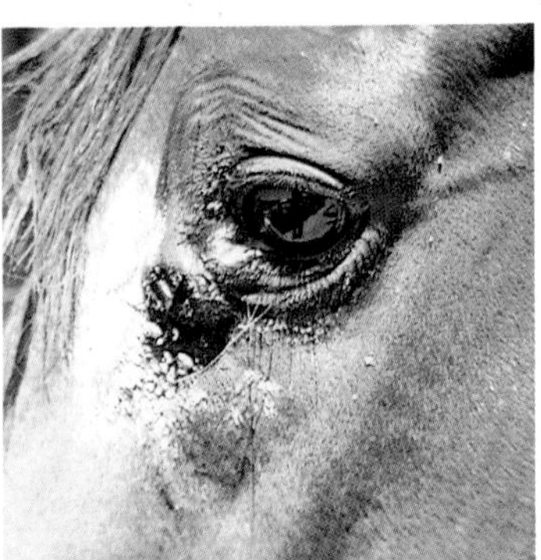

Possible diagnosis: Summer Sores (Habronema Infestation) – *see page 285*

Habronema infection in the eye region

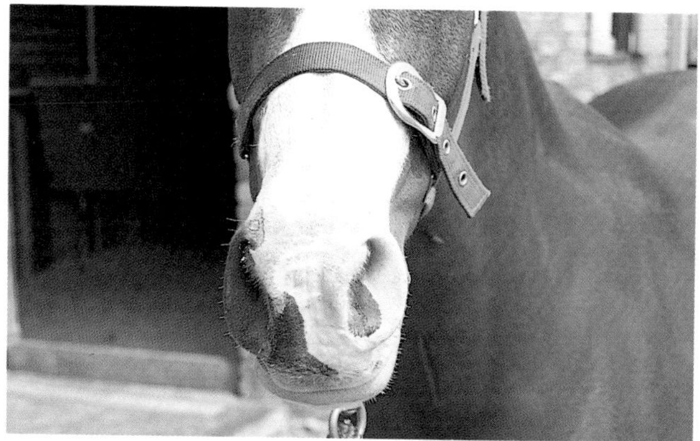

Sunburnt nose

► Hairless, non-pigmented areas such as nose become red, swollen, and ooze serum – skin often peels – leaves raw, bleeding area – very sensitive to touch. Along back of horse serum mats with hair, dries, hardens and peels – after long period skin becomes dry and wrinkled, with little or no hair cover.

Possible diagnosis: Sunburn – *see page 285*

---

► Lumps vary in size from 2 mm to 2 cm – pink to grey in colour – common sites are nose, lips, eyelids and cheeks – lumps are raised with rough horny surface.

Possible diagnosis: Warts – *see page 296*

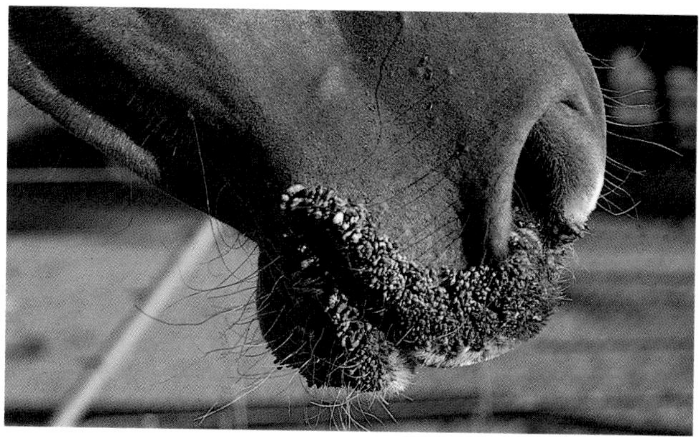

Warts around the lips

# TEETH PROBLEMS

Find below the group of associated signs that best fits what you observe in your horse.

BACKGROUND

The horse uses its incisor (front) teeth to pick, tear or cut grasses and pasture when grazing, and the molar (back) teeth for grinding and masticating food in preparation for digestion. We can use the horse's incisor teeth to tell its age accurately up to 8 years; thereafter the degree of accuracy decreases.

## ASSOCIATED SIGNS

► Slow eating – excessive salivation – quidding food i.e. dropping partially chewed food from mouth – masticating food difficult.

Possible diagnosis: Dental Caps – *see page 194*

---

► Horse refuses food – slow in eating – excessive salivation – blood coming from mouth – quidding food i.e. dropping partially chewed food from mouth – lack of response to the bit such as pulling or hanging to one side – throwing head – loss of condition – swelling of cheeks which are painful to pressure.

Possible diagnosis: Lacerated Cheeks and Tongue – *see page 232*

---

► Horse has one or two extra incisor teeth – sometimes a complete second row of teeth.

Possible diagnosis: Supernumerary Teeth – *see page 286*

---

► Upper and lower incisors do not meet – lower jaw is too short.

Possible diagnosis: Undershot Jaw – *see page 293*

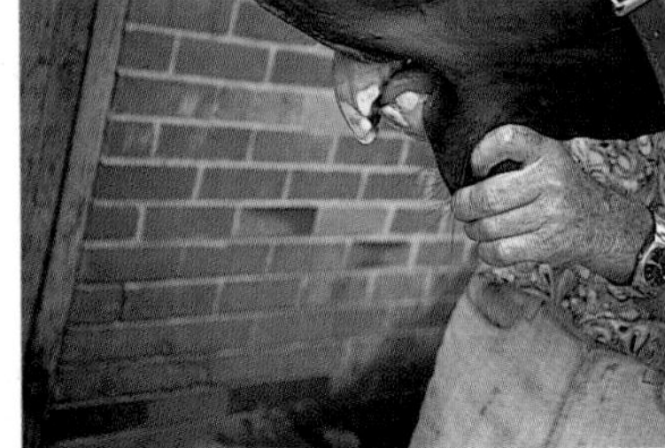

Parrot mouth (undershot jaw)

# TEMPERATURE

*Find below the group of associated signs that best fits what you observe in your horse.*

## BACKGROUND

Refer to the earlier section 'Signs of a Healthy Horse' for the method of taking a horse's temperature and reading the thermometer.

The normal temperature of a horse ranges from 37.7°C to 38.6°C, although it may be slightly higher in very hot climatic conditions or after strenuous exercise. The temperature of young horses (weanlings) is normally slightly higher than that of mature horses. Otherwise, an elevated temperature indicates an infection. A sub-normal (low) temperature is often a danger sign that the horse's defence mechanisms have given up the fight against an overwhelming infection. In such cases, contact your veterinarian immediately.

## ASSOCIATED SIGNS

► Swelling can be seen or felt under skin – when forming in early stages, swelling is diffuse, hot, painful, hard – later stages more localised, softer, less painful, forms a point – at this stage when pressed with finger it usually shows a depression – horse may be lethargic, off food, have temperature.

Possible diagnosis: Abscess – *see page 154*

---

► Foetal membranes (afterbirth) hanging from mare's vulva for more than 8 hours.

Possible diagnosis: Afterbirth, retained – *see page 155*

---

► Vary according to route of infection – generally there is high temperature, severe depression, diarrhoea and abdominal pain, followed by swelling under jaw, on chest, abdomen and in lower limbs – death follows in 2–4 days.

Possible diagnosis: Anthrax – *see page 158*

---

► Temperature high – may be up to 41.5°C – dull – unsteady – swelling of limbs and trunk – blood in urine – anaemic – presence of ticks – occurs mostly in tropics and sub-tropics where conditions suitable for survival of tick – may be fatal.

Possible diagnosis: Babesiosis – *see page 162*

---

► Found in Germany – more common among horses 3–6 years of age – lethargy – chewing slowly, eventually unable to chew or swallow – compulsive circling – skin becomes hypersensitive. Signs worsen progressively over 1–3 weeks leading to death in 70–90% of cases.

Possible diagnosis: Borna Disease – *see page 166*

---

► Difficulty in grasping food with lips and teeth – drools saliva – unable to drink – paralysis of tongue – slow mastication – unable to swallow – wobbliness in fore and hindquarters – knuckling over – stumbling – collapse with constant paddling movements of limbs leading to death.

Possible diagnosis: Botulism – *see page 167*

---

► *Horse*: Dung is cow-like, porridge-like – discoloured watery fluid. Signs of discomfort when passing motion – swishing tail – looking at flank – tucking up abdomen.
*Foal*: Dung fluid, putrid – straining – tucking up abdomen. Can cause death.

Possible diagnosis: Diarrhoea – *see page 195 (horse); page 196 (foal)*

---

► Encountered mainly in tropics and sub-tropics.

Early stage: swelling of penis and prepuce – scrotum and testicles become swollen – male and female genitalia are covered with blisters, pustules and ulcers.

Later stage: weakness of hindquarters – knuckling – stumbling – circular swellings of skin on croup, shoulder, chest and abdomen – 2–4 cm in size – appear and disappear rapidly.

Terminal cases: hypersensitive to touch – ticklishness and paralysis of hindquarters – severe weight loss – unable to get up.

Possible diagnosis: Dourine – *see page 196*

---

► Pale gums and conjunctiva (inside eyelids), sometimes yellow with jaundice – not eating – weight loss – weakness – fluid swelling under belly and in legs – clear discharge from eyes and nose.

Possible diagnosis: Equine Infectious Anaemia – *see page 200*

---

► Dry cough – discharge from both nostrils – initially clear and watery – progressing to thick mucus – loss of appetite – lethargy.

Possible diagnosis: Equine Influenza – *see page 201*

---

► Pregnant mares may abort during illness or shortly after – incubation period of 2–6 days – symptoms may be high temperature (42°C) – off food – dopey – weak – inflamed, discoloured eyes – nasal discharge. Some show oedema (swelling) in legs, udder and underbelly – constipation – colic – diarrhoea.

Possible diagnosis: Equine Viral Arteritis – *see page 202*

---

► Incubation period of infection about 2 weeks – symptoms of a cold – nasal discharge – coughing – sneezing – respiratory disease – abortion may occur up to 4 months after infection when mare appears healthy – abortion usually occurs from 5th month onwards. Foetus expelled rapidly with placenta – virus can affect brain and spinal cord of mare causing paralysis of hindquarters – foetus aborted after 6 months shows discolouration of placental fluid and hooves due to diarrhoea in uterus. Disease found throughout world including Australia.

Possible diagnosis: Equine Viral Rhinopneumonitis – *see page 202*

---

► Swelling on one or both sides of withers – hot to touch – painful – may erupt discharging straw-coloured fluid – in few days discharge changes to whitish-yellow pus.

Possible diagnosis: Fistulous Withers – *see page 203*

---

► Young foals with purulent discharge from both nostrils – rattling sound in chest – coughing – laboured breathing – often stimulated by handling – harsh coat – elevated temperature.

Possible diagnosis: Foal Pneumonia (Rattles) – *see page 204*

---

► Nasal discharge – weight loss – coughing – rapid shallow breathing – hear moisture in chest – ulcerations of nasal cavity and skin – often erupting on inside of hock – nodules under skin are up to 2 cm in diameter and discharge a honey-like pus.

Possible diagnosis: Glanders – *see page 216*

---

► Discharge from one or both nostrils depending on whether one or both guttural pouches are involved – often nasal discharge obvious when horse puts head to ground. Swelling below ear, on one or both sides – where head meets neck – discomfort – breathing difficult. When tapped with fingers swelling may be firm, containing pus (infected).

Possible diagnosis: Guttural Pouch, Infected – *see page 217*

---

► Jaundice (yellow discolouration of mucous membranes of conjunctiva and gums) – may be accompanied by high temperature – not eating – depression. Skin of white horses may show signs of yellowing.

Possible diagnosis: Hepatitis – *see page 223*

---

► Vaginal discharge – failure to conceive or maintain pregnancy – reproductive cycle normal.

Possible diagnosis: Infected Uterus – *see page 226*

---

► Lethargic – dull – not eating or eating a little – no other signs.

Possible diagnosis: Infection of Unknown Origin – *see page 228*

---

► Heat, pain and swelling in affected joint(s) of new-born foal – lameness – stiffness in movement – temperature rise.

Possible diagnosis: Joint ill – *see page 229*

► Udder may be larger on one side than other – painful to touch, hot, swollen, hard, sometimes lumpy – milk may be thick and discoloured – may have temperature.

Possible diagnosis: Mastitis – *see page 239*

---

► Mild lameness shortly after shoeing – generally worsens each day – 3–7 days after being shod, horse is acutely lame, just touching ground with toe of foot – hoof wall is warm to touch – pastern may be swollen – arteries on either side of pastern supplying hoof pulsate more rapidly and strongly than normal. When squeezed with hoof testers (pincers) or tapped with hammer, severe pain exhibited by horse pulling foot away – pain is worse when pressure is applied over offending nail.

Possible diagnosis: Nail Prick – *see page 240*

---

► Acute stage: swelling of scrotum – stiff gait – one or both testicles may be involved – hot and painful if palpated – may refuse to serve mare (breed) – may have temperature rise.

Chronic stage: testes may be of normal size – insensitive to touch – feel harder than normal.

Possible diagnosis: Orchitis – *see page 243*

---

► Temperature rise – disinclined to move – reluctant to lie down – grunting associated with breathing – abdominal muscles tense – loss of appetite and weight – dehydration.

Possible diagnosis: Peritonitis – *see page 260*

---

► Discharge from both nostrils – off food – lethargic – rapid shallow respiration – cough – high temperature – breath may have foul odour – hear moisture in chest as horse breathes in and out – doesn't want to move or lie down – nostrils may be flared.

Possible diagnosis: Pneumonia – *see page 261*

---

► Tenderness around poll – painful, well-defined, or a diffuse, ill-defined swelling may be seen – stiffness in head movement – pus discharge in mane – may be noticed when putting on bridle.

Possible diagnosis: Poll Evil – *see page 263*

---

► Symptoms arise 12–24 hours after foaling – temperature rise – lethargy – off food – bloody brown or creamy yellow discharge from vulva – constant drip of blood – laminitis (see page 211) may be evident.

Possible diagnosis: Post-Foaling Metritis – *see page 263*

---

► Found in Europe and US – early signs: drooling of saliva – spastic lip movement – hyperexcitable – leading to depression and not eating. Rare cases become aggressive (biting and kicking). Paralysis develops – first affecting the ability to swallow and vocal cords (altered whinny) – then spreads to hindquarters with collapse and death in 2–7 days after initial signs.

Possible diagnosis: Rabies – *see page 268*

---

► Foal shows signs of depression 12–24 hours after birth – strains repeatedly to urinate – very little or no urine passed – straining can be similar in constipated foal – do not confuse.

Possible diagnosis: Ruptured Bladder – *see page 273*

---

► Copious, purulent discharge from both nostrils – loss of appetite – slight cough – lymph nodes under jaw inflamed and swollen – laboured respiration.

Possible diagnosis: Strangles – *see page 283*

---

► Stiffness – rigidity of whole body – third eyelids partially cover the eyes – difficulty with taking food into mouth and chewing – drooling a mixture of saliva and food – general stiffness leads to convulsions and death in up to 80% of cases.

Possible diagnosis: Tetanus – *see page 288*

# VICES

Find below the group of associated signs that best fits what you observe in your horse.

BACKGROUND

Horses in herds once roamed freely in a natural environment seeking natural pastures. Today, no matter how large the stable, it is small and lonely compared to the open range. Often a vice is purely the result of boredom and solitary confinement.

Vices serve no useful purpose; the horse may cause damage to property, to itself or other horses, or to persons nearby. Vice may be related to the horse's basic genetic temperament or to poor management, metabolic disturbance, excessive energy, boredom or loneliness.

## ASSOCIATED SIGNS

► Horse grasps solid object with incisor teeth – arches neck – gulps air.

Possible diagnosis: Crib Biting (Wind Sucking) – *see page 189*

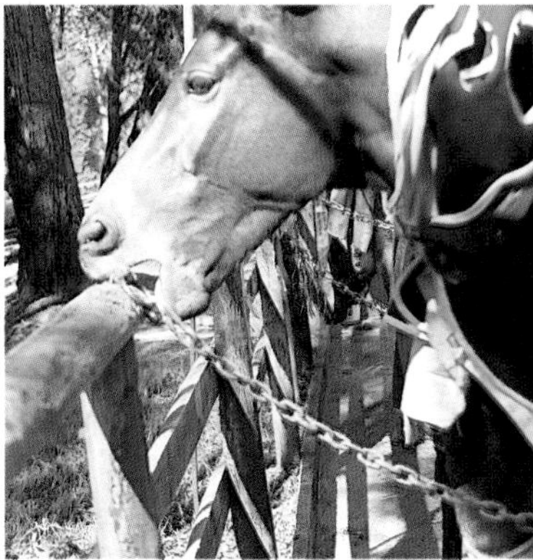

Wind sucking

► Kicking, e.g. stable doors and tailgates of floats – rearing with flailing legs – striking – turning round, presenting hindquarters with one leg raised as warning – pulling away – laying back ears, extending neck and showing teeth ready to bite.

Possible diagnosis: Kicking – Striking – Biting – Rearing – Pulling Back – *see page 295*

► Horse constantly paws ground – digs large holes, mostly near doorways – toe of hoof worn.

Possible diagnosis: Pawing – *see page 258*

---

► Horse constantly walks in circles around stable – often wears deep track in earthen floor.

Possible diagnosis: Stall Walking – *see page 283*

---

► Horse swings head and neck from side to side – alternates weight on front legs with each swing.

Possible diagnosis: Weaving – *see page 297*

---

► Chewed timber doors, fences and stable walls.

Possible diagnosis: Wood Chewing – *see page 300*

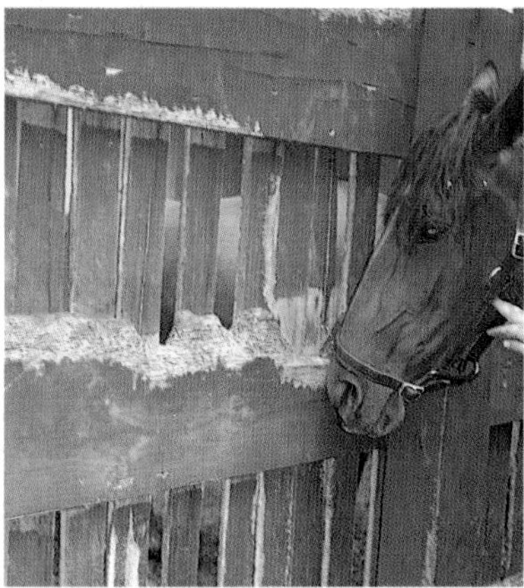

Wood chewing

# WORMS (PARASITES)

## ASSOCIATED SIGNS

- Weight loss – dull harsh coat – pot belly – pale mucous membranes of eyelids and gums – diarrhoea – tail rubbing – poor appetite – reduced performance – poor stamina – colic – coughing in young foals – botfly eggs on coat.

*Possible diagnosis: Parasites (worms) – see page 248*

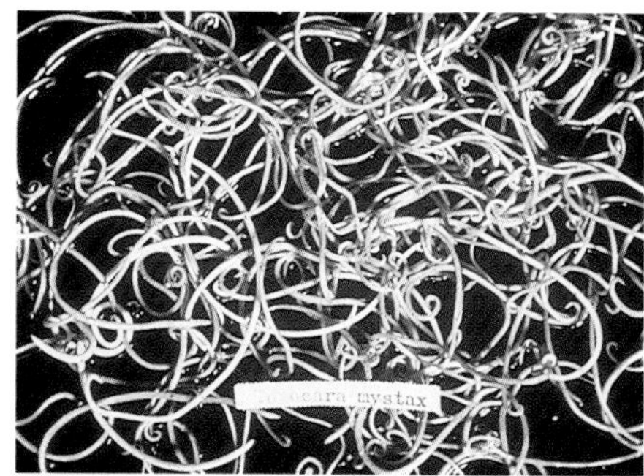


Roundworms

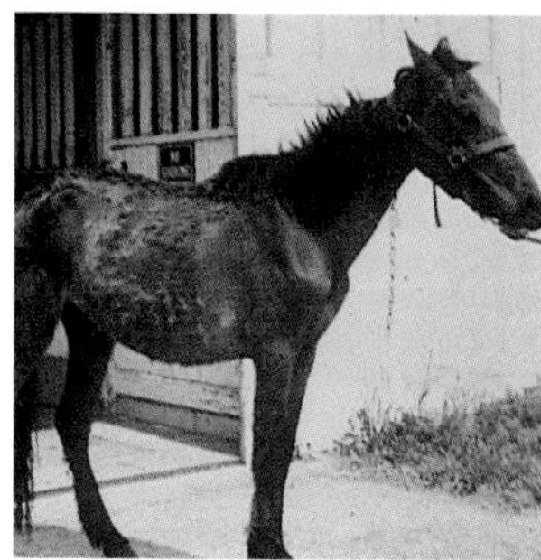

Typical signs of worms: weight loss and a dull harsh coat

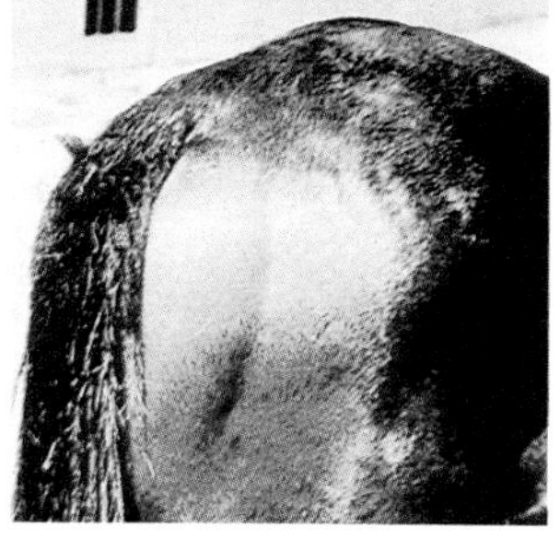

Tail rubbing, caused by irritation from worms, has removed all the hair

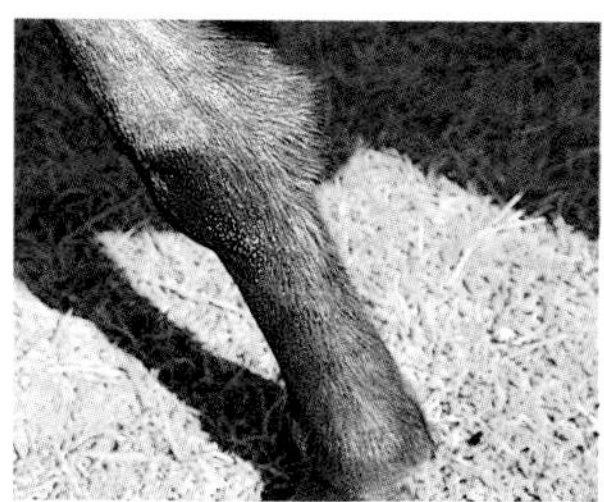

Bot eggs on the leg

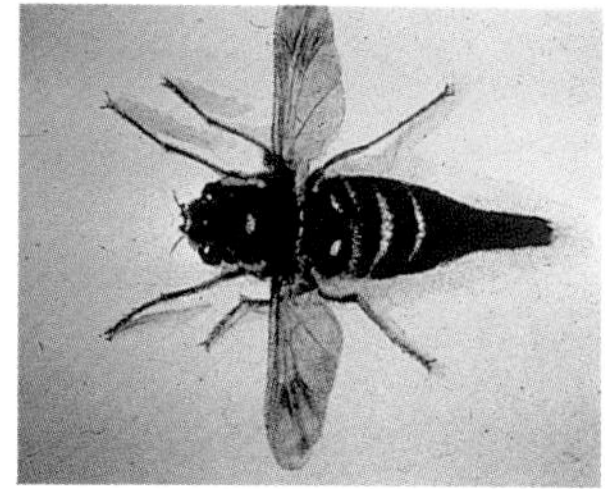

Botfly

# WOUNDS

Find below the group of associated signs that best fits what you observe in your horse.

## BACKGROUND

The horse is susceptible to infection. Most wounds are contaminated, so consult a veterinary surgeon about tetanus injection and treatment with antibiotics.

## ASSOCIATED SIGNS

► Hair and surface layer of skin removed – painful to touch – bleeds a little – often contaminated with grit and dirt.

Possible diagnosis: Abrasion – *see page 154*

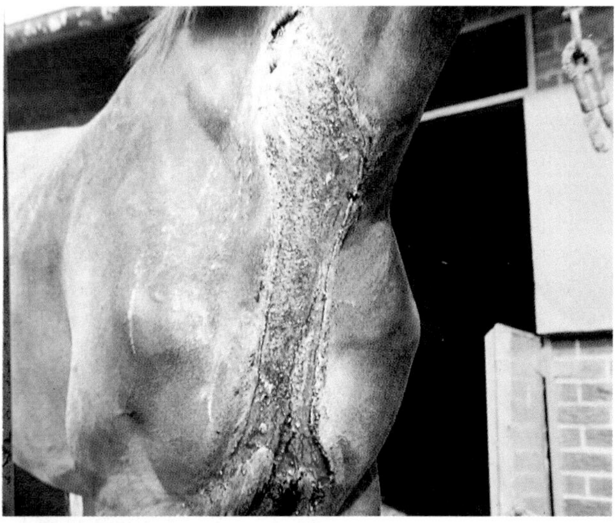

Extensive wound requiring a skin graft for complete healing

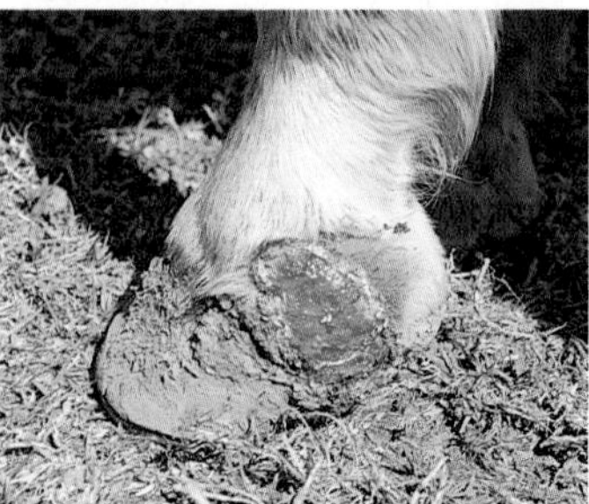

Abrasion of coronary band and skin just above hoof

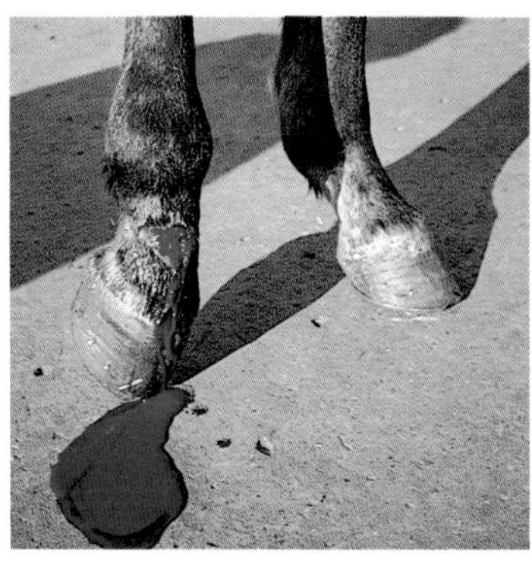

Abrasion haemorrhaging

---

► Bruising and swelling of skin and underlying tissues – skin may or may not be broken.

Possible diagnosis: Contusion – *see page 187*

---

► Edges clean cut – fairly well opposed – minimum of tissue damage.

Possible diagnosis: Incised Wound – *see page 300*

---

► Wound edges irregular – jagged and gaping – sometimes whole sections of skin and underlying tissue torn away – not usually acutely painful – bleeding varies depending on which blood vessels are severed.

Possible diagnosis: Laceration – *see page 233*

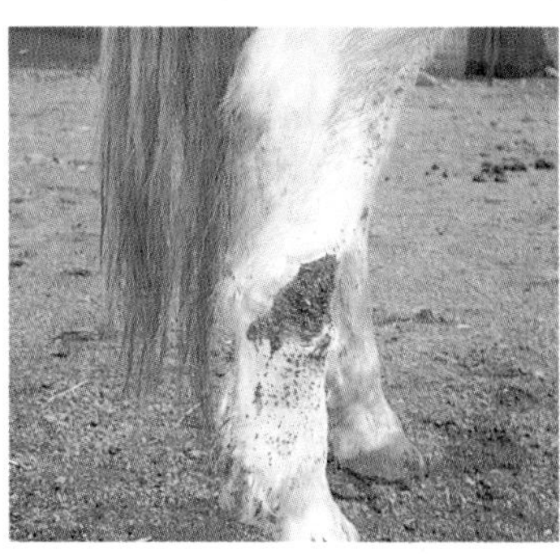

Laceration caused by barbed wire

► Hole in sole of foot or skin – variable size – neat or ragged edge – variable tissue damage under skin – may or may not be bleeding.

Possible diagnosis: Puncture Wound – *see page 265*

# YELLOW GUMS & CONJUNCTIVA

Find below the group of associated signs that best fits what you observe in your horse.

## ASSOCIATED SIGNS

► Incubation period 8–14 days – varies according to whether disease is acute or chronic.

Acute: temperature over 40°C – weakness – wobbly – muscle tremor – yellow, inflamed mucous membranes – fluid swelling (oedema) under belly and legs – exercise produces pounding heartbeat – anaemia develops later – usually continues eating – death may occur.

Chronic: weight loss – poor performance – exhaustion – severe anaemia – horse may recover, attacks occurring less frequently – or can die unexpectedly in acute relapse. Horses that apparently recover remain carriers of virus.

Possible diagnosis: Equine Infectious Anaemia – *see page 200*

---

► Jaundice (yellow discolouration of mucous membranes of conjunctiva and gums) – may be accompanied by high temperature – not eating – depression. Skin of white horses may show signs of yellowing.

Possible diagnosis: Hepatitis – *see page 223*

---

► Occurs in new-born foal – sluggish – dull – weak – no longer suckles – lies down – rapid, shallow breathing (panting), especially after exercise – anaemic (pale gums and conjunctiva) – then gums and conjunctiva change to varying shades of yellow – after 24 hours urine dark brown – may collapse and enter coma.

Possible diagnosis: Isoimmune Haemolytic Jaundice – *see page 228*

# TREATMENT OF DISEASES AND HEALTH PROBLEMS A–Z

Here you will find diseases and problems listed alphabetically, with details of signs, causes and treatments.

# INDEX OF TREATMENT OF DISEASES

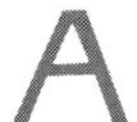

# ABORTION: Bacterial

SIGNS
Usually occurs before 150th day of pregnancy but possible at any stage – premature birth of foal – may be unable to suck – weak and dull – often retention of placenta and vaginal discharge.

CAUSE
Numerous types of bacterial infection – most common is a streptococcal infection – the different types can be differentiated by swabs, culture and selective staining – mares running with cattle may pick up Brucella – if associating with pigs may pick up leptospirosis.

TREATMENT
Some infections can be prevented by the veterinarian taking a swab, doing a culture, then giving mare appropriate antibiotic – all this to be done while mare is in season but before she is served. Some cases are given uterine irrigation with saline antibiotic solution.

# ABORTION: Fungal

SIGNS
Occurs about 10th month of pregnancy – swab and culture by veterinarian will show signs of fungi if present.

CAUSE
Fungus.

TREATMENT
Veterinarian will administer appropriate treatment.

# ABORTION: Hormonal

SIGNS
May occur between 3rd and 5th month – low levels of hormone, progesterone, known to cause abortion at certain stages of pregnancy – mare may have history of abortions unrelated to infection or other causes.

CAUSE
Inadequate level of progesterone.

TREATMENT
Veterinarian evaluates blood level of progesterone – if necessary administers progesterone therapy.

# ABORTION: Stress

SIGNS
Severe stress – excitement – depression – dehydration – weakness – weight loss.

CAUSE
Transporting over long distances – deprivation of food and water over long periods – trauma – excessive, vigorous, lengthy exercise, e.g. endurance ride.

TREATMENT
Avoid above causes especially between 90th and 160th day of pregnancy.

# ABORTION: Twinning

SIGN
Abortion of two foetuses – most common between 5th and 9th months.

CAUSE
One foetus develops more rapidly than the other – assumes most of mother's blood supply – other foetus dies – abortion of both.

TREATMENT
Mares with history of twins should be examined by veterinarian when in season and before being served, to evaluate size and number of follicles on ovaries – allow mare to be served only when one follicle larger and more mature than any other. Twins can be diagnosed by ultrasound or rectal palpation – veterinarian can terminate one or both pregnancies according to position in uterus.

# ABORTION: Viral

## (a) Equine Herpes I (Equine Viral Rhinopneumonitis)

SIGNS
Incubation period of infection about 2 weeks – symptoms of a cold – temperature up – nasal discharge – coughing – sneezing – respiratory disease – abortion may take place up to 4 months after infection when mare appears healthy – abortion usually occurs from 5th month onwards. Foetus expelled rapidly with placenta – virus can affect brain and spinal cord of mare causing paralysis of hindquarters – foetus aborted after 6 months shows discolouration of placental fluid and hooves due to diarrhoea in uterus. Disease found throughout world including Australia.

CAUSE
Virus enters horse through respiratory tract – in the young and weak causes bronchitis and pneumonia – some cases carry the virus without symptoms – virus spread by direct contact – droplets from sneezing, coughing, feeding, drinking – contact with aborted foetus or its membrane – if group of pregnant mares infected with virus you have an abortion epidemic.

TREATMENT
None specific – antibiotics – rest – isolate new mares for 3 weeks – isolate aborted mares – burn or bury aborted material – disinfect stalls and abortion area with Formalin – keep weanlings some distance from brood mares – vaccination in US and UK – contact your veterinarian.

## (b) Equine Viral Arteritis

SIGNS
Pregnant mares may abort during illness or shortly after – incubation period of 2–6 days – symptoms may be high temperature (42°C) – off food – dopey – weak – inflamed, discoloured eyes – nasal discharge. Some show oedema (swelling) in legs, udder and underbelly – constipation – colic – diarrhoea.

CAUSE
Virus worldwide but not in Australia – transmitted by direct contact – droplets from sneezing, coughing, eating – nasal discharge – saliva.

TREATMENT
Rest for 1 month after signs disappear – alter diet – if constipated feed bran mash – if diarrhoea dry feed – isolate infected horses, stalls and grazing area – disinfect stable area – contact your veterinarian for antibiotics – eye ointment – electrolytes and fluids – good immunity persists after natural infection.

# ABRASIONS

SIGNS
Hair and surface layer of skin removed – normally painful to touch – a little haemorrhage – often contaminated with grit and dirt.

CAUSE
Hair and surface skin removed by friction – contact with brick wall, rope, hard ground, gate, floats, etc.

TREATMENT
Remove dirt and foreign material by hosing wound with firm pressure of water – pressure not too severe as may drive foreign material further into wound – an alternative is to clean wound with peroxide – foaming action helps to flush out dirt – also germicidal. When wound clean – pat dry with clean gauze – dust with antibiotic powder – or paint with gentian violet – or use aerosol pack containing antibiotic and triple dye. Leave abrasion open – if blood oozing freely, cover with gauze bandage – if abrasion large do not exercise horse until healing obvious.

# ABSCESS

An abscess is a collection of pus enclosed in a capsule in the tissues under the skin.

SIGNS
Swelling seen or felt under skin – when forming in early stages swelling is diffuse, hot, painful, hard – in later stages more localised, softer, less painful, forms a point – at this stage when pressed with finger it usually shows a depression – horse may be lethargic, off food, have temperature.

CAUSES
In most cases a foreign body penetrates skin and underlying tissue, e.g. when rubbing neck against fence horse may cause splinter of wood to penetrate skin – when grazing may pick up grass seed in cheek – when walking in yard nail may puncture foot.

Abscesses under jaw usually caused by internal infection such as strangles – internal abscesses sometimes develop on liver, lungs and elsewhere – associated with generalised bacterial infection.

TREATMENT
In early stages, if puncture site obvious – thoroughly cleanse area with iodine-based scrub or Hibiclens – remove dirt, debris or dead tissue – check wound to see no foreign body remains embedded. Apply hot foment to area – smear a drawing agent,

such as Magnoplasm, over the swollen area – call your veterinarian who will administer antibiotics and anti-tetanus vaccine. Treatment may cause forming abscess to subside and tissue to return to normal.

If abscess points, your veterinarian will lance it for drainage – wound should be kept open while drainage is taking place. If large pocket exists after pus drained out – irrigate twice daily by squirting a syringe full of peroxide into cavity. Aid drainage by gently pressing from outer extremities of abscess towards opening. Continue treatment till opening almost closed.

# AFTERBIRTH (retained)

The afterbirth may be expelled from the mare before she gets to her feet after foaling. On average it is expelled within 3 hours but may hang from the mare's vulva for up to 8 hours.

## SIGNS

Afterbirth has not come away from the mare within 8 hours of foaling.

## TREATMENT

Risk of mare treading on membranes (afterbirth) and tearing them with hind feet – best to tie membranes in a knot – prevent it dragging on the ground. Contact your veterinarian.

Afterbirth may be easily removed by manually pulling on it with firm, even tension – if afterbirth doesn't give way – stop pulling – you could cause haemorrhage, damage to lining of uterus and infection due to membranes tearing and remaining in uterus. Use of drugs often necessary to aid in separation of afterbirth from attachments in uterus – other drugs are used to prevent laminitis (founder).

Once afterbirth removed – important to lay out the membranes on ground – check that all afterbirth has been expelled – if small portion is retained in uterus, could lead to serious complications such as infection and founder.

# ANAEMIA: due to bleeding

External bleeding is easily recognised. Internal bleeding is more difficult to diagnose but should be considered after severe accidents, e.g. falls.

## SIGNS

Bleeding – pale conjunctiva (membrane inside eyelid) – pale gums – weakness.

CAUSE
Trauma – blood vessel ruptured due to weakened blood vessel wall (parasitic aneurysm).

TREATMENT
*Internal:* if suspected, call your veterinarian.
*External:* first step control bleeding – if blood oozing, apply direct pressure to site with piece of clean gauze or sheeting – don't dab or wipe – tends to promote bleeding – hold pressure on wound for 10 minutes – remove pressure – evaluate wound – if bleeding recommences apply further pressure.

If blood flowing freely – apply gauze wad or suitable absorbent material to wound with heavy pressure from clean hand – wrap firmly but not tightly 75mm wide Elastoplast over wad of gauze – leave in place for 30 minutes – remove bandage and gauze wad – evaluate wound – do not use cotton-wool – fibres tend to act as foreign body in wound – slow down healing process.

If arterial bleeding – blood bright red, spurts out with pulsating action – apply heavy pressure with gauze wad in hand over wound site. Wrap firmly 75mm wide Elastoplast bandage over gauze wad – this applies pressure and immobilises edge of wound – helps stop bleeding – keep horse calm, preferably tied up in stall – any movement will stimulate circulation and hence bleeding – call veterinarian for further advice.

If horse bleeding from inaccessible area, e.g. nostrils – restrict movement – hose site with cold water or apply ice pack in towel – call your veterinarian. Tourniquets not recommended. Don't watch your horse bleed to death – keep horse calm – apply direct pressure.

# ANAEMIA: due to nutritional deficiency

Definite diagnosis can be made only by a blood count.

SIGNS
Pale mucous membranes – dull harsh coat – weight loss – poor performance – poor appetite – reduced stamina.

CAUSE
Dietary deficiency – iron, copper, cobalt.

TREATMENT
Iron fumurate 1–2 g daily with vitamin B12 and anabolic steroids. Iron injections given to horse only if it has extremely low haemoglobin and red cell levels. Injection of iron dextran preparations associated with fatal reactions, especially if course of injections given.

# ANAEMIA: due to stress

Anaemia is not a disease, it is a symptom of something else, so it is essential to find the causal factor(s) before treatment is initiated. Anaemia is reduced levels of haemoglobin and red blood cells to below normal, affecting the oxygen-carrying capacity of the blood and resulting in poor performance. A stressed horse, e.g. one in hard training and performing regularly, will readily show signs of anaemia. On the other hand, an unstressed horse with anaemia may not show any signs.

SIGNS
Lethargy – loss of appetite – restlessness – loss of condition – poor coat – poor performance. Colour of tissue around eye (conjunctiva) and gums reflects status of red blood cells in horse – normal colour is pink – white indicates severe anaemia – in many cases the colour does not fall into either category.

CAUSES
Continual hard work – exercise on track – racing – leads to stress – depresses erythropoesis, i.e. red blood cell production – exacerbating this problem is increase in red blood cell fragility and destruction – horses that cannot cope with stress become anaemic.

TREATMENT
No treatment should be initiated till cause diagnosed – blood count essential for accurate diagnosis – treatment best left to your

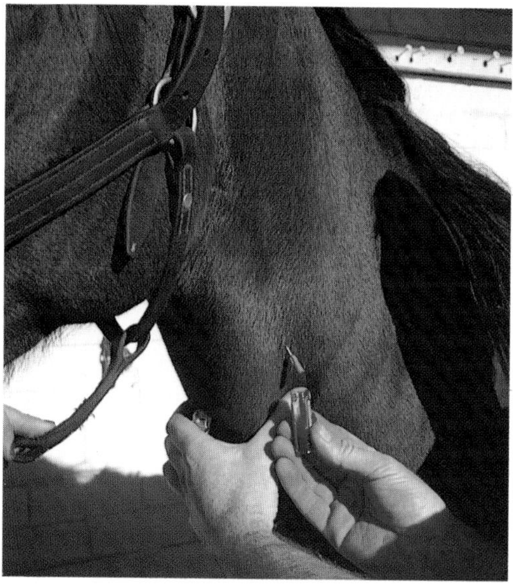

Taking blood for a blood count

veterinarian. Some cases of anaemia can be avoided by good nutrition and good worming program.

As a rule, all performance horses should be on a selected, well-balanced vitamin and mineral supplement – concentration of vitamins and minerals should be fully stated on container – an iron supplement that will directly influence haemoglobin levels is recommended – keep in mind that some irons are not readily absorbed.

# ANHYDROSIS (Dry Coat; Inability to Sweat)

SIGNS

Anhydrosis is inability to sweat – observed in horses in tropical countries – more commonly found among horses imported from temperate zones – within few weeks horse sweats less – sweating may be confined to localised areas – crest of neck – under chest – skin dry, inelastic and flaky – very high temperature after exercise (43°C) – severe respiratory distress – may affect horse born in tropics.

CAUSE

Failure of sweat glands to operate – due to permanently high blood adrenalin level.

TREATMENT

Air conditioning and cooling of stables – work horses in cool of early morning – hose down afterwards. Provide electrolytes in diet. If horse doesn't respond move to cooler climate. Some success achieved by administration of drugs – contact your veterinarian.

# ANTHRAX

A very acute disease caused by the bacterium *Bacillus anthracis*. It occurs all over the world, affecting all animals including humans.

SIGNS

Vary according to route of infection – generally there is a high temperature, severe depression, diarrhoea and abdominal pain, followed by swelling under jaw, chest, abdomen and in lower limbs – death follows in 2–4 days.

CAUSE

Bacteria in suitable conditions can survive in soil for 40 years – enter body by ingestion, inhalation or through a break in skin.

TREATMENT
Contact your veterinary surgeon immediately – isolate horse from all other animals while waiting – if horse dies, do not attempt a post-mortem – seek advice from appropriate authorities regarding disposal of body and disinfection.

# ARTHRITIS

Arthritis is inflammation of a joint (which is made up of bones, cartilage, ligaments and joint capsule). The joint capsule produces fluid that lubricates the joint.

SIGNS
Swelling localised in joint(s) – in initial stage (acute) may be firm, warm, swollen, painful to touch – with time (chronic stage) becomes hard – often not warm to touch – less painful – may be restricted movement of joint – eventually permanent joint damage.

CAUSES
Trauma that may be due to kick, cut, fall or penetrating foreign body – infection entering joint through wound or localising in the joint from general infection – poor conformation placing abnormal stress on a joint or joints – poor nutrition, e.g. lack of calcium.

TREATMENT
Treatment varies according to cause – call veterinary surgeon – best able to diagnose arthritis and pinpoint cause. While waiting for veterinary surgeon, apply pressure bandage to affected joint – immobilise horse by putting it in stable or tying it up – cold hose the joint and pack it with ice if there are no obvious signs of infection – an antiphlogistine poultice will help reduce swelling.

Chronic arthritis varies in its response to liniments, anti-inflammatory agents and radiation therapy.

# ATRESIA ANI

SIGNS
Foal cannot pass motion – straining – appears constipated – becomes colicky – no anal opening.

CAUSE
Born with no opening at site of anus.

TREATMENT
See veterinarian – condition corrected surgically.

# AZOTURIA (Tying-Up)

Years ago this condition was called Monday morning disease because draught horses, pit horses and other working horses in good, well-muscled condition exhibited symptoms on Monday mornings after they had rested over the weekend and had been fed a high-grain diet. The condition is characterised by stiffness, pain and muscle tremor involving the muscles of the hind-quarters, except in severe cases where the muscles of the fore-quarters may be involved as well. Tying-up is a less severe form of azoturia.

## SIGNS

Vary widely – in mild cases, during or after exercise, horse steps short in hind limbs, giving appearance of stiffness – in severe cases, horse will show stiffness, pain, sweating and muscle tremor – the stiffness, involving both hind limbs and front limbs, may progress to point where horse cannot move and may lie down – affected muscles are very hard to the touch, indicating cramp – urine may vary in colour from dark brown to reddish-black, according to severity of condition.

## CAUSES

Horses worked at irregular intervals and fed high-grain diets are most susceptible to azoturia. Ingested grain is converted to glycogen, which is stored in muscles and elsewhere – if horse rested for periods of 1–2 days while on high-grain diet, large quantities of glycogen are stored in muscles – glycogen is used by muscles as source of energy when work is being done – waste product from chemical change that takes place is lactic acid – if large volume of glycogen is stored, a large volume of lactic acid is produced when horse exercises – if lactic acid cannot be expelled from muscle tissue, it damages muscle fibres, causing condition known as tying-up – if large areas of muscle fibres are damaged or even destroyed, azoturia results.

Some horses not on grain diets tie up because they are hypersensitive to lactic acid or their particular metabolism does not cope with it efficiently.

## TREATMENT

Stop exercising horse when you notice that it is tying up – in all cases, except severe ones, walk horse for 30 minutes – if it appears no better, call your veterinary surgeon – walking aids circulation of blood to muscles with consequent removal of lactic acid, thus helping to prevent severe cramping.

The veterinarian can confirm the condition not only by its history and clinical signs but also by taking blood count and doing certain serum enzyme tests.

Keep horse warm by seeing it is well rugged – tempt it with fluids containg electrolytes which, if drunk in any quantity, will help to flush out kidneys. With aid of information gained from blood count, the veterinary surgeon can administer a muscle relaxant, diuretics, tranquillisers and anti-inflammatory agents if required, as well as specially prepared fluids and electrolytes by stomach tube or intravenous methods.

All grain should be eliminated from diet and horse should be offered bran mash as mild laxative – horses susceptible to frequent tying-up should have low-level grain diet – normally grain level in diet should be in proportion to amount of work done – e.g. if in any one week a horse works for six days, followed by a day off, reduce quantity of grain in feed for that day.

Exercise horse every day, even if it is just walking exercise and consult your veterinary surgeon about regular use of a particular vitamin supplement as a preventive measure.

Recovery can take place within hours, though in severe cases it may take weeks.

# B

## BABESIOSIS (Piroplasmosis)

This disease is transmitted by ticks and is confined to tropical and sub-tropical zones.

SIGNS
Incubation period 6–21 days – high temperature, up to 41.5°C – dull – unsteady – swelling of limbs and trunk – possible blood in urine – jaundice (yellowing mucous membrane of eyes and gums) – ticks on horse – if horse survives it develops chronic state and slowly loses weight – remains anaemic.

CAUSE
Species of tick – pathological tests conducted by veterinarian to identify.

TREATMENT
Good general nursing – medication prescribed by veterinarian – immunity develops following infection – re-infection appears necessary for maintenance of immunity.

## BIG HEAD

SIGNS
Shifting lameness – reluctant to move – lying down – swelling around jaw and cheeks in severe cases.

CAUSE
General cause calcium phosphorus imbalance – can be brought about by horses grazing on pasture predominantly tropical grasses (buffel grass and setaria) – these grasses contain oxalates which bind calcium in the intestine – prevents absorption of calcium through intestinal wall – or by horses being fed diets high in phosphorus such as high-grain diets.

TREATMENT
Calcium deficiency or calcium phosphorus imbalance can be diagnosed by blood test or urinalysis.

To prevent and treat, remove horse from the pasture – or add feed supplement of 1 kg rock phosphate mixed with molasses – horses on high-grain diets should be given 40 g calcium carbonate daily.

# BIRTH DIFFICULTIES

A mare's labour usually proceeds without problems but, if complications occur, it is important to recognise them early and take quick knowledgeable action. The wisest course is to get in touch immediately with a veterinarian. Sometimes owners try to cope with complications themselves and worsen them or create others.

## SIGNS

Mare straining in labour – obvious contractions and straining – after about 25 minutes no foal appears.

After 15 minutes of obvious straining and contractions – mare appears to give up – in following half hour her efforts weak and less frequent.

No obvious contractions – mare continually getting up and down – showing signs of pain by kicking, swishing her tail, looking at flanks.

Other signs are one leg of foal presented – excessive bulging of mare's anus – forefeet presented but head turned back in uterus – foal lying on back with soles of feet and lower jaw uppermost – foal doubled on itself so head, forefeet and hind feet all presented together – hind feet presented first with soles facing upwards – buttocks, tail, points of both hocks presented – buttocks and tail of foal presented (breech) – twin foal.

## CAUSES

Mare's pelvic canal too small – foal too big – dead foal – twins – abnormal presentation – hormonal imbalance in mare.

## TREATMENT

To examine foal presented at vulva – hands and arms should be scrubbed thoroughly – surgical gloves should be worn – mare's anus and vulva should be washed down with non-irritant antiseptic, e.g. Hibiclens.

If normal straining and normal presentation – no foal expelled – take hold both forelegs – gently but firmly pull downwards and outwards – if no change call your veterinary surgeon.

If only one leg presented – make sure your hand and arm is well scrubbed with non-irritant disinfectant – wear surgical glove if possible – lubricate bare arm or glove – place hand, arm into vagina – feel gently for other leg – avoid irritating and/or bruising mucous membrane which may then swell or become infected – if foal's elbow caught on brim of mare's pelvis – pull leg out to bring it almost level with other leg in normal position – this action lifts foal's elbow over pelvic rim – allows free passage of foal.

Excessive bulging of mare's anus may indicate feet of foal pushed towards mare's rectum by her contractions – if continues may tear recto-vaginal wall – fistula results and mare may be rendered infertile – to prevent, place hand inside vagina – guide foal's feet to vaginal opening.

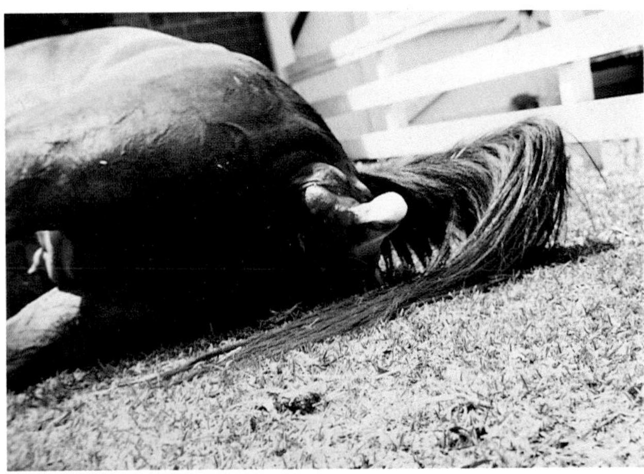

One leg of the foal is presented

More complex cases need help of veterinary surgeon, e.g. – forefeet presented but head back in uterus resting on foal's flank – foal on its back with soles of forefeet and lower jaw uppermost – foal doubled on itself so head, forefeet and hind feet presented together – hind feet presented first, soles facing upwards – buttocks and tail of foal are presented (breech presentation) – buttocks, tail, both points of hocks presented – twin foals – foal is born dead.

Veterinary surgeon should also be called immediately – if no foal appears after about 25 minutes of contraction and straining – if no obvious contractions and mare continually getting up and down, showing signs of pain by kicking, swishing tail and looking at flanks – if after 15 minutes of obvious contractions and straining mare gives up, her efforts for next half hour weak and less frequent.

# BLEEDER (Epistaxis)

This term is not used for the equine equivalent of human haemophiliacs. Bleeding is a condition common to racehorses. A bleeder is potentially dangerous to itself, to its rider and to other horses and riders in the field. During races there have been cases of horses bleeding severely, collapsing and bringing down others in the field. Some owners and trainers have argued that the bleeding was caused by the nose hitting the ground when the horse collapsed. This argument has been refuted by film showing blood streaming from the horse's nostrils before its collapse.

SIGNS
Obvious sign is horse bleeding from one or both nostrils after race, track work or sometimes swimming – bleeding may begin during exercise, immediately after, or sometimes hours after exercise has finished – blood may lie inside nostrils, drip to ground, or flow freely. Some horses bleed in the lungs – only signs of this may be laboured breathing, distress and coughing – often the more serious type of haemorrhage.

CAUSES
Bleeding can be due to defect in blood-clotting mechanism, high blood pressure or fragile capillaries in nose or lungs.

TREATMENT
Contact your veterinarian as this problem can be fatal. He can evaluate defect in clotting mechanism by taking blood sample and doing specific tests for clotting. Using an instrument called a rhinolaryngoscope he can examine nasal passages, throat and upper windpipe to see if a ruptured vessel in any of those areas is causing haemorrhage. Various drugs can be used to harden fragile capillaries, reduce blood pressure and rectify deficiency in clotting mechanism. Rest is essential for any capillary rupture to heal properly. Feeding horse at ground level, thus making it put its head down to eat, may help strengthen capillaries in nostrils.

# BOG SPAVIN

Bog spavin is associated with inflammation of the joint capsule. In many cases, the swelling is merely an unsightly blemish which has little or no effect on the usefulness of the horse.

SIGNS
Soft fluid-filled swelling on upper and inner side of hock – more often than not, no heat, pain or lameness.

CAUSES
Faulty conformation such as straight, upright hock, producing abnormal strain on joint capsule – sudden, sharp movements commonly met in such activities as polo, jumping and calf roping stretching and tearing the joint capsule of the hock.

TREATMENT
In early phase acute cases treated with cold hosing, rest, immobilisation by stabling, application of pressure bandage. In chronic cases, treatment by veterinarian – can vary from blistering to draining fluid and injecting anti-inflammatory agent into joint capsule.

# BONE SPAVIN

Bone spavin is caused by arthritis of the bones in the area of lower, inner side of the hock. Some horses with obvious bone spavin show few or no signs of lameness; others may be very lame with no signs of swelling. Horses with bone spavin may still be useful, although fluctuating lameness may recur at varying intervals.

SIGNS
Hard bony enlargement felt and seen on lower and inner side of hock – horse lame when cold – lameness characterised by reduced flexion of hock and shortening of stride in affected leg – often disappears as horse warms up with exercise – sometimes worsens.

CAUSES
In many cases due to poor conformation, such as sickle and cow hocks – poor conformation usually inherited. Condition can also be caused by stress and strain placed on hock through participation in such activities as polo, calf roping and racing, especially by young horses.

TREATMENT
Accurate diagnosis important to determine severity of condition – this, in turn, will determine type of treatment. Your veterinary surgeon with aid of X-rays will make diagnosis.

He may advise any one of a number of treatments or a combination of them. One is to rest horse in spelling paddock for minimum of 6 weeks after corrective trimming and shoeing – the toe of the foot should be rasped square – shoe with raised heel and rolled square toe should be fitted – causes leg to move in a straight line rather than deviating outwards, thus alleviating strain on inside of hock.

Other treatments are radiation, anti-inflammatory agents, or surgery to sever section of tendon that runs over the spavin.

# BORNA DISEASE

SIGNS
Found in Germany – more common among horses 3–6 years old – lethargy – chewing slowly, eventually unable to chew or swallow – compulsive circling – skin becomes hypersensitive. Signs progressively worsen over 1–3 weeks leading to death in 70–90% of cases.

CAUSE
Virus which affects central nervous system – incubation period of 2–3 months – first recognised in Germany almost 200 years ago.

TREATMENT
No vaccine is available – disinfecting stable, feed bins, etc. with formalin may help to prevent spread of virus. Death often results from pneumonia – mortality rate 70–90%.

# BOTULISM

Botulism is the technical term for forage poisoning. It does not occur very often, as its cause (feeding on mouldy hay or chaff or on grain contaminated by vermin) is widely known and avoided.

SIGNS
Difficulty in grasping food with lips and teeth – drooling saliva – inability to drink – paralysis of tongue – slow mastication – inability to swallow – wobbliness in fore and hindquarters – knuckling over – stumbling – collapse with constant paddling movements of limbs leading to death.

CAUSE
Botulism is brought about by ingestion of food or water contaminated by bacteria (*Clostridium botulinum*) that multiply and produce their toxin or poison.

TREATMENT
Mortality rate from botulism is high so contact your veterinary surgeon immediately. While waiting, treat horse for shock (see page 37). Vaccines are available but they are seldom used because of infrequency of disease in horses.

# BOWED TENDON

A tendon is a tough, sinewy tissue attaching muscle to bone. It is made up of numerous fibrils and surrounded with a tendinous sheath. Those involved in the condition known as bowed tendons are the superficial and deep flexor tendons, located in all four legs behind the cannon bone, running from knee to fetlock. The tendons more commonly involved are those in the front legs.

Bowed tendon is very common in racehorses, often causing premature retirement. The bow is caused by swelling fibrils, oozing inflammatory fluid, and by capillary haemorrhage. The size of the bow varies according to the number of fibrils stretched or torn and the position of the injury. You can get some idea of the stress placed on the flexor tendons if you consider the force of the impact when a horse with a body weight of about 500 kg lands on one leg, galloping, say, at 60 k/hr.

Recovery from a bowed tendon is more likely with modern advanced treatment. However, unless the tendon is returned to its original state, any weakness in the form of a damaged bowed tendon is likely to show up under extreme stress, such as in racing.

## SIGNS

Swelling located in any one of the legs, mainly a front leg, behind cannon bone, running from knee to fetlock. In early stages: swelling – heat – pain on pressure – may step short or be severely lame – in later stages: swelling reduced and localised, leaving hard fibrous bow in tendon.

## CAUSES

Many predisposing factors – conformation (long sloping pasterns), shoeing (long toe and low heel), fast gaits, forced training (unco-ordinated leg movement due to fatigue), excessive demand (the horse at full gallop or trot is asked to give that 'little bit extra'). External damage may cause bowed tendon – usually brought about by blow from another foot.

## TREATMENT

Contact your veterinarian – while awaiting arrival, apply cold to swollen tendon in form of running water from hose for 30 minutes. Running water has gentle massaging effect on tendon. Alternatively, pack ice in towel and hold over swelling – or bandage it with cotton-wool soaked in iced water. Following the cold treatment – wrap cotton crepe bandage firmly and evenly around leg from just below the knee to fetlock joint – leave bandage in place unless leg swells, causing further excessive pressure – if it does, remove bandage and reapply.

Immobilise horse by putting it in the stable with deep bed of straw or other suitable bedding – if tendon grossly swollen, immobilise horse further by tying it up – rest most important. Do not exercise horse, even if swelling is only minor, until veterinary opinion has been sought.

If farrier available in early phase of tendon sprain, have horse shod, shoe having raised heel to reduce tension on tendons.

Veterinary treatment of bowed tendon varies according to the cause. May involve: rest only – spelling in a paddock from 6–12 months – administration of antiphlogistic, anti-inflammatory and/or internal sclerosing agents – tendon splitting – tendon transplant – recently developed technique of carbon filament implant.

# BRITTLE HOOVES

SIGNS

Dry, brittle hooves - cracks in wall - pieces of wall breaking away.

CAUSES

Dry weather conditions with horse confined on a dry hard surface - excessive rasping of hoof wall.

TREATMENT

Aim is to return moisture to hoof wall which will soften and regain its elasticity - also to prevent moisture being lost from hoof wall. Glossy surface on hoof wall is called the periople - reduces rate at which moisture evaporates from wall - excessive rasping of wall at time of trimming or shoeing destroys periople - causes hoof wall to dry out.

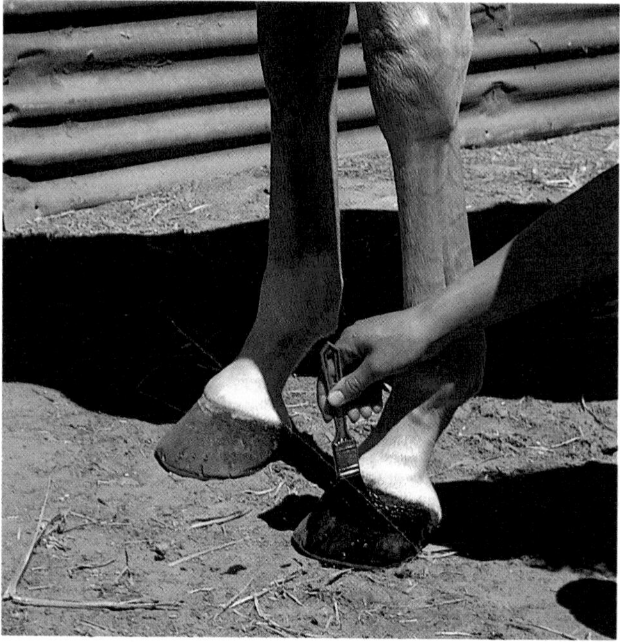

Painting the hoof wall

Paint wall and sole of hoof with a mixture of one-third stockholm tar, one-third neatsfoot oil and one-third sump oil daily. For treatment of cracks see hoof crack, page 223.

# BRONCHIAL ASTHMA (Allergic Bronchitis)

This condition is common in horses kept in stable complexes. In its chronic form it is also known as heaves.

SIGNS
Clear watery discharge from both nostrils – persistent hacking cough – clear watery discharge from eyes – may be normal between bouts of coughing attacks.

CAUSES
Hay and grain dust – straw bedding – mouldy food – mites in hay – stabling with poor ventilation. Precipitating cause may be an upper respiratory viral infection.

TREATMENT
Good quality hay fed damp to settle dust – good quality straw bedding dampened to keep dust down or change to peat bedding – stable should be well ventilated – if possible put horse in yard or paddock during day – give regular exercise but not on dusty tracks.

Contact your veterinarian who can advise and treat horse with antihistamines, anti-allergy medications.

Remember: if horse allergic to environment, allergy will recur once treatment ceases if environment not changed.

# BRUISED SOLE

SIGNS
If you clean sole with a hoof knife, bruising will be evident by presence of blood under the surface – if bruising severe, horse will show signs of lameness and react to pressure on sole.

CAUSES
Sharp stones or exercise on hard, uneven ground that damages the toe or quarter areas of sole.

TREATMENT
In case of mild bruising rest and time will allow blood to disperse – in severe bruising, sole over bruised area should be cut away with clean knife to provide drainage – apply tincture of iodine to the opening, as well as a drawing agent (magnesium sulphate) – cover bruised area with a bandage to prevent further contamination – an E–Z boot may also be used. Your veterinarian should be called to administer a tetanus injection – if bruise is infected or in danger of becoming infected, antibiotics will also be administered.

# BRUSHING

SIGNS
Inside edge of foot in motion touches inside of fetlock of opposite leg – may occur with forelegs or hind legs.

CAUSES
Poor conformation such as turning out or turning in from fetlock – poor co-ordination associated with fatigue.

TREATMENT
Toe of offending foot trimmed square and hoof shod with square-toed shoe to make foot break in a straight line – inside branch of shoe rolled and set slightly in from border of inside (medial) wall to reduce chance of interference – as a protective device, bandage fetlock of leg that is being hit or fit brushing boot.

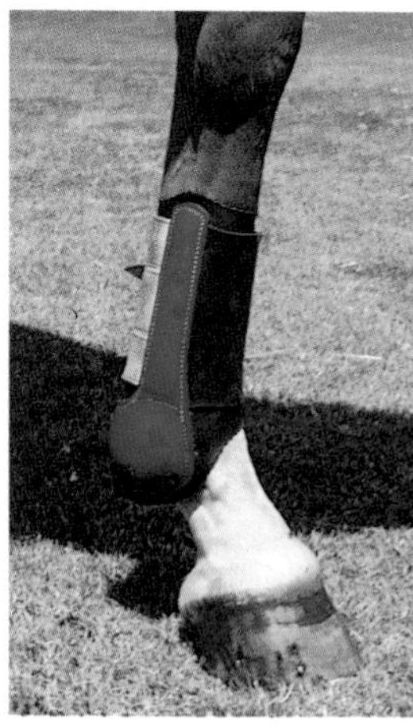
A brushing boot

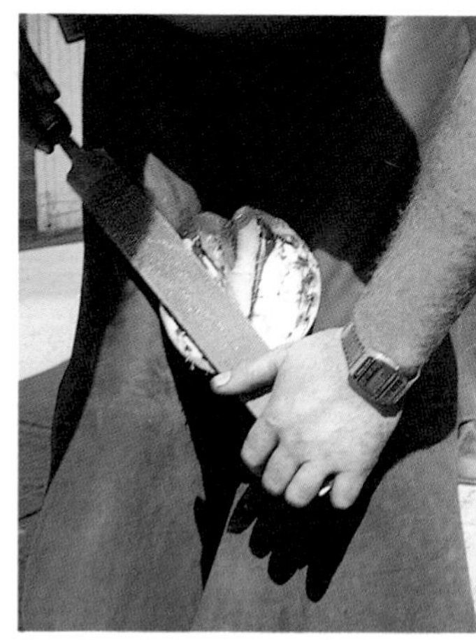
Rasping the toe square

# BURNS

Often burns in horses are not like the classic burns in humans where the skin is red and swollen, leading to formation of blisters.

## SIGNS

Blackened hair – swelling of skin and underlying tissues – blisters on the skin – dead skin – sloughing of the skin leaving large denuded areas which ooze a clear or light-coloured fluid. Depending on area of skin involved the horse may be tender in local areas – reluctant to move – generally in pain – in a state of shock if extensive areas involved.

## CAUSES

Bush, grass and stable fires – electrical burns from lightning strike – chemical burns – rope burns.

## TREATMENT

Depends on area, depth and position of burn. Burns where skin has been devitalised are very susceptible to infection. Call your veterinarian – he will administer antibiotics and possibly corticosteroids. Apply antibiotic ointment to burn – cover with a sterile bandage – change dressing every 2–3 days. Provide horse with electrolytes in drinking water.

Healing facilitated by immobilisation – tying up – stabling – bandaging – plaster cast. If horse mutilating itself use tranquilliser and neck cradle as preventive measure.

If more than 50% of horse's surface area is involved, euthanasia is recommended.

# C

## CANCER (Squamous Cell Carcinoma)

Squamous cell carcinoma is one of the most common forms of skin cancer in the horse.

SIGNS
Swelling with or without ulceration – often involves third eyelid (nictitating membrane), eyelids and penis.

CAUSE
Unknown.

TREATMENT
Your veterinarian will make definite diagnosis by biopsy and pathological examination – surgery followed by radiation treatment often successful.

## CAPPED ELBOW (Shoe Boil)

SIGNS
Round, soft, fluid-filled swelling on point of elbow – up to 10 cm in diameter – most cases not sore to touch – lameness slight and temporary if present.

CAUSES
When horse lying down with front legs curled under, one of its front shoes may hit or press on point of elbow. Or shoe on foot of affected limb of horse with very flexible joints and flamboyant action may also hit point of elbow while in motion.

TREATMENT
In early stages: cold compresses (ice wrapped in a towel) – cold hosing – reduction of exercise to walking – may be sufficient to

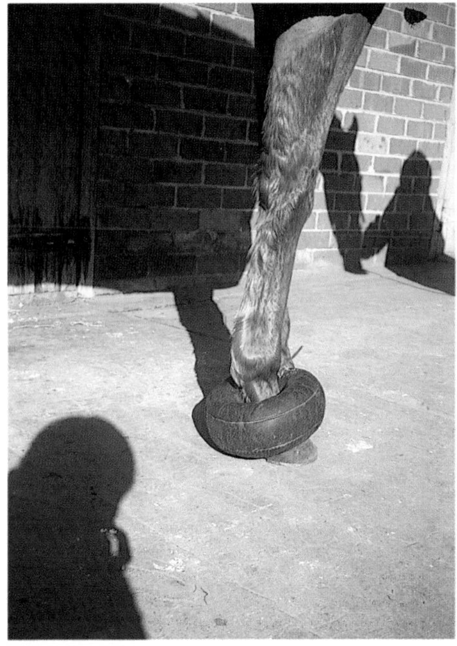

A special padded leather roll protects the elbow

reduce swelling. If it persists for 3–4 days or becomes larger, call your veterinarian – he will drain fluid and inject drug into lump to prevent refilling. Preventive measures: specially padded leather roll strapped around the pastern while horse in stable will protect elbow when horse lies down – horse hitting elbow when in motion, corrective trimming and shoeing indicated.

# CAPPED HOCK

Horses in confined spaces such as stables, horse floats or trailers are susceptible to capped hock. To prevent it, remove the horse from stable to yard or paddock if it is a kicker.

SIGNS
Swelling on point of hock – in early stages round, soft, fluid-filled, up to 10 cm in diameter – not sore to touch – lameness, if present, slight and temporary. Old swellings filled with fibrous tissue – hard to the touch.

CAUSE
Most common cause – kicking, rubbing or striking the point of hock against hard object.

TREATMENT
In early stages: cold compresses (ice wrapped in a towel) – cold hosing – reduction of exercise to walking – may be sufficient to reduce the swelling. If swelling persists for 3–4 days or becomes larger, call your veterinarian – he will drain fluid and inject anti-inflammatory agent into lump to prevent refilling.

# CARPITIS

This is inflammation of the knee joint.

SIGNS
Horse lame – swelling in localised circumscribed area of knee or more generalised – recent swellings soft – older swellings may be very hard – flexibility of knee restricted – signs of pain when knee bent.

CAUSES
Concussion associated with such activities as racing, polo, jumping, hunting and eventing – trauma due to kick from another horse, or horse pawing at stable door hitting front of its knee. Forced training of immature horses and poor conformation are other causes.

TREATMENT
Swelling, if soft, is due to excess production of joint fluid from joint capsule – if hard, swelling may be due to fibrous tissue, arthritic spurs (new bone growth) or fracture of one of small bones in knee. Call veterinary surgeon to X-ray knee to determine exact cause of swelling. Treatment may involve one or more of the following: draining the joint – rest – injecting an anti-inflammatory agent into the joint – pressure bandage – blistering – pin firing – surgery – radiation therapy.

If horse not lame and knee has soft swelling – owner should rest horse for 14 days – cold hose knee for 20 minutes twice a day – apply a pressure bandage. If swelling still evident or horse sore at end of 2 weeks, seek opinion of veterinary surgeon.

# CATARACT

The lens is the area of the eye surrounded by the pupil. Cataract is crystallisation of the lens. The bluish cloudy appearance that the lens of a horse's eye develops with advancing age is not to be confused with a cataract.

### SIGNS

In immature cataracts lens partly or wholly cloudy but allows some light to pass through – some sight is present. A mature cataract is dense, silvery-white and fills entire pupil, which is usually dilated. Light cannot penetrate opaque lens, thus total blindness in that eye. A cataract can form in one or both eyes.

If horse totally blind in both eyes, it will walk into walls and other objects – often subjecting itself to severe abrasions. If horse totally blind in one eye, it will often walk into objects on that side – when approached on its blind side horse will often jump with fright when touched. If horse partially blind in one or both eyes, it may shy or balk at objects unnecessarily – may have difficulty in negotiating objects when the light is subdued, as at dusk.

### CAUSES

Congenital – trauma – infection – chronic inflammation of the eyeball.

### TREATMENT

Once cataract starts to form, treatment cannot prevent its further development – when it has reached maturity it can be removed surgically and horse's sight is restored.

## CHOKE

### SIGNS

Distressed – refuses to eat – extends its head and neck – salivates – coughs – grunts – paws the ground – agitation gives way to depression. Food and saliva regurgitated through nostrils – lump may be seen and felt on left side of neck.

### CAUSE

Occurs when oesophagus obstructed by food or foreign body – horses that bolt feed or with teeth abnormalities more susceptible when fed dry grains – boluses administered orally may lodge in oesophagus – foreign bodies often responsible, e.g. wire, nails, pieces of wood.

### TREATMENT

Call your veterinarian – try to determine cause while waiting – do not allow horse to drink – may be taken into lungs and cause pneumonia. Solid objects more serious as blockage than grain, hay, grass. If lump felt in neck – according to position – gently, firmly massage it up or down.

Preventive measures – for greedy horses place few large stones in feed bin – put hay in hay net – check horse's teeth every 6 months for abnormalities – horses prone to choke on dry grains change to boiled grains.

# CHRONIC OBSTRUCTIVE PULMONARY DISEASE

See Bronchial Asthma (page 170).

# COITAL EXANTHEMA

SIGNS
Small blisters first on head, then on body, of penis – blisters develop into pustules – then into ulcers in few days. Further use of stallion will result in extensive damage to penis surface with subsequent loss of libido.

CAUSE
Herpes virus – transmitted during service (sexual intercourse).

TREATMENT
Rest from service for at least 10 days until ulcers have healed completely. Contact your veterinarian, who will supply antibiotic cream to apply to penis every second day.

# COLIC: Flatulent

SIGNS
Pain not as severe as spasmodic colic – more continuous – horse dull – paws ground – makes frequent attempts to urinate – may or may not lie down – seems afraid to do so – abdomen enlarges noticeably in upper right flank – breathing may be interfered with – small amounts of dung and gas passed.

CAUSE
Formation of large volumes of gas mainly in large intestines – due to excess feeding on lush green pasture, clover, other legumes.

TREATMENT
Call veterinarian – may treat condition by administering 5 litres paraffin oil with stomach tube – in more acute cases may be necessary to puncture bowel using trocar and cannula inserted into right side of flank.

# COLIC: Gastric Dilatation

Horse will have a history of eating large quantities of wheat, maize, coarse straw, young clover, mouldy grain or hay; greedy overfeeding.

SIGNS

Severe abdominal pain – swollen abdomen when tapped with fingers has a drum-like sound and feel – horse kicks at abdomen – throws itself on ground – rapid panting-type breathing – sweats profusely – mucous membranes around eyes and gums vary from brick red to bluish colour – breath is sour – horse may adopt dog-sitting position – vomiting rare. If stomach ruptures – horse quietens down – its temperature falls – goes into shock – can die suddenly.

CAUSE

Distension of stomach due to greedy overfeeding of large quantities of wheat, maize, coarse straw, young clover, mouldy grain or hay – large volumes of gas produced, causing distension – this in turn causes muscles around inlet and outlet of stomach to close, preventing escape of food and gas – as stomach distends, more fluid from stomach lining pours into stomach, further aggravating the distension.

TREATMENT

Contact your veterinarian immediately – be careful handling horse as it will sometimes react violently – veterinary surgeon will tranquillise and administer pain-relieving drugs – immediately horse is manageable stomach tube is passsed down to allow gas, fluid and food material to escape – important action is to alleviate distension of stomach as quickly as possible – if veterinarian cannot be contacted, carefully administer orally 5 litres of paraffin oil.

Even if horse appears to recover call your veterinarian because laminitis (founder), see page 211, often follows gastric dilatation.

# COLIC: Impaction

SIGNS

Symptoms usually develop slowly – abdominal pain may disappear for day or two – reappears more violently. Horse dull – passes dung in small quantities, drier and harder than usual – looks at flanks – restless – lies down – characteristic pose lying on side – legs and head extended – occasionally raising head to look at flank – may lie on side for 5–15 minutes – rises – goes down again – in some cases frequent straining to pass urine.

CAUSE

Impaction of small and large intestines – constipation – due to feed being eaten hurriedly (bolting of food) or intake of excess low-grade roughage making intestinal digestion difficult – large bolus forms, leading to impaction.

TREATMENT
Call your veterinarian – will administer paraffin oil via stomach tube – softens impacted mass – rectal massage sometimes breaks down mass allowing movement to take place.

Prevent horses bolting feed – place large stones in manger – allows small mouthfuls at a time – put hay in a net or hayrack – do not use straw as a bedding if horse eats it.

# COLIC: Obstruction

SIGNS
Violent pain – restless – paws ground – looks at flanks – kicks out violently – throws itself on ground – rolls violently – rapid respiration, heart rate, pulse rate – sweating – dehydration – as shock sets in mucous membranes of gums and eyes turn brick red to bluish to white – no gut sounds. As death approaches – less violent – legs and ears cold – may be free from pain.

CAUSES
Various causes such as foreign body – twisted bowel – strangulated intestine resulting from hernia – intussusception (telescoping of one section of bowel inside another section of bowel).

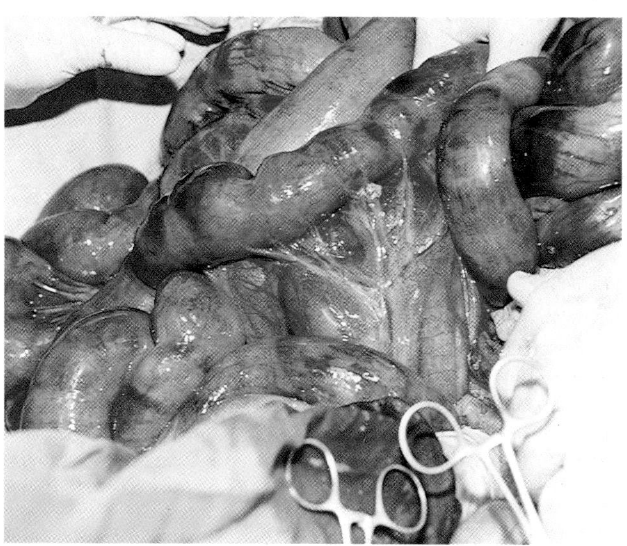

A twisted bowel

TREATMENT
Urgent – contact your veterinarian – time of utmost importance to give best chance of survival – veterinarian's examination will

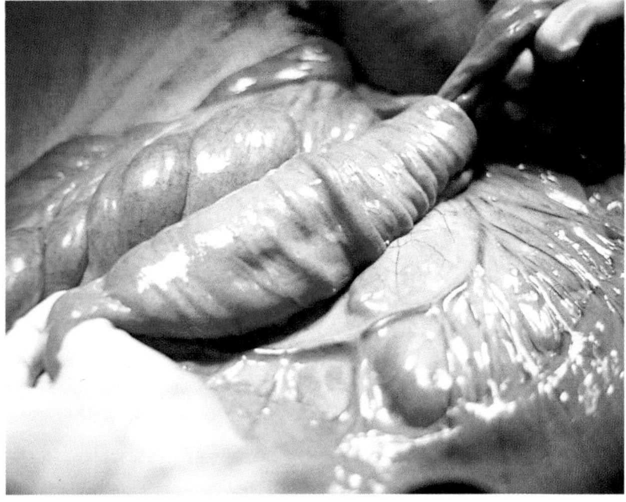

Intussusception: this kind of colic requires emergency veterinary attention

cover pulse, heart and respiration rates – intestinal sounds – blood count – rectal examination – paracentesis (puncturing abdominal cavity with needle to collect peritoneal fluid for examination).

# COLIC: Spasmodic

SIGNS

Sudden, severe pain followed by interval of calm – paws the ground – stamps hind feet – kicks at belly – crouches as if to lie down – looks at flanks – stretches as if to urinate – penis may be extended. As attack progresses pain attacks more frequent and longer – horse may throw itself down – roll – jump up again – generally violent. Frequent, rapid, loud intestinal sounds heard.

CAUSES

Pain caused by strong rapid contraction of muscles in intestinal wall. If teeth neglected – develop razor sharp edges – severely lacerate inside of cheeks, gums, tongue – horse finds it difficult to grind feed – poorly digested feed upsets intestinal motility – leads to spasmodic colic.

Hypermotility or speeding up of gut movements can be caused by excitement – exhaustion – overwork – migrating

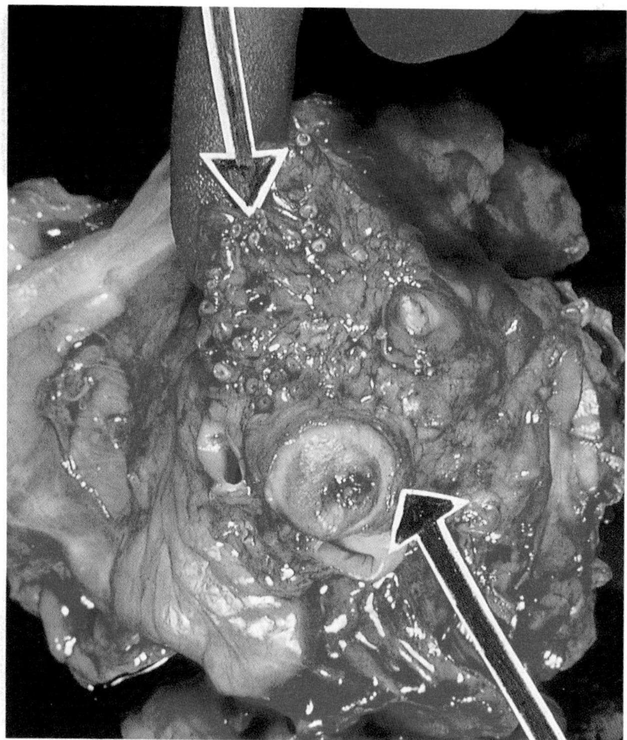

Verminous aneurysm caused by migrating red worm larvae

immature red worm larvae (*Strongylus vulgaris*). Spasmodic colic often early sign of small intestine obstruction.

## TREATMENT

Contact veterinarian immediately – drugs will stop spasm of intestine and alleviate pain – while waiting walk your horse to ease pain and to prevent injury – if legs and ears cold (shock), rug horse. Preventive measures: adopt correct worming procedures and check teeth with view to rasping every 3 months.

# CONJUNCTIVITIS

The conjunctiva is the membrane lining the inside of the eyelid around the eye and can be seen when the upper or lower eyelid is pulled away from the eyeball. Conjunctivitis is inflammation of the conjunctiva.

## SIGNS

Conjunctival membrane is very red, swollen and moist – discharge – varies from copious amounts of clear, watery fluid that runs down cheek to thick, yellow-green pus that lies in corner of eyelids, sometimes matting them together – one or both eyes may be involved – if both eyes, cause is often a viral infection or allergy.

## CAUSES

Foreign bodies such as chaff, dust or grit, or mud in the eye – infection (bacterial and viral) – eye injury.

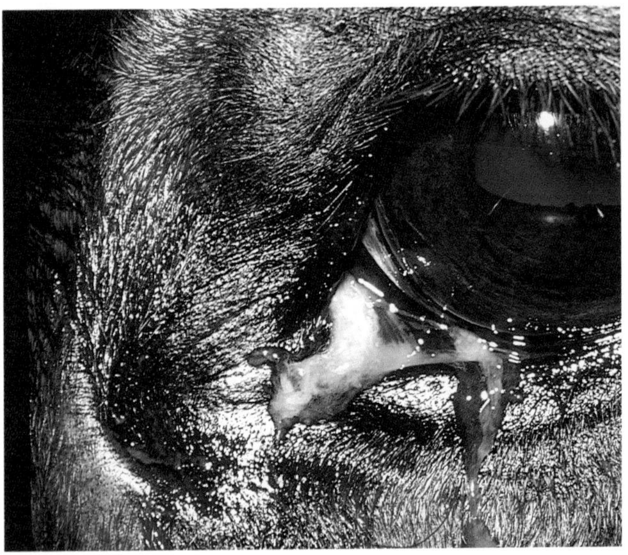

*Conjunctivitis: a mucus discharge*

## TREATMENT

Call your veterinary surgeon – other complications are often associated with conjunctivitis, such as ulceration of the surface of the eyeball – if incorrectly treated, may lead to permanently damaged eye or blindness.

While waiting for veterinarian to arrive – bathe eye for 10

minutes four times a day with water that is not too hot f( hand, wiping away discharge adhering to the eyelids – if po keep horse in dust-free environment – out of the wind – ( direct sunlight. If foreign body present in conjunctiva – rem , provided that it can be done readily – if not, leave eye alone – you may increase irritation of conjunctiva and even damage eyeball itself.

There are many different types of eye ointments, each of which has a specific purpose. Eye ointments should not be used indiscriminately for conjunctivitis because some can make certain conditions worse.

# CONSTIPATION (foal)

SIGNS

Most obvious signs 12–18 hours after birth – straining with restlessness – tail cocked – with more frequent straining less suckling – may cease if pain continues – with no relief abdominal pain becomes more severe – foal gets up and down – lies flat out – rolls on its back – crouches – throws itself to ground – thrashes violently – ultimately goes into state of shock – veterinary help needed to save foal. Occurs more frequently in colts than in fillies.

CAUSE

Most common cause in young foal – blockage of bowel by meconium – thick, dark, tar-like faeces in lower bowel at time of birth. Condition may be worsened by swelling of rectum and anus, thus narrowing opening through which motion passes.

TREATMENT

If you don't see foal's meconium passed, give it an enema within 12 hours of birth – if meconium passed but later foal strains with no sign of motion – wise to give it an enema – take care not to damage lining of rectum and anus – about 300 ml of warm, mild, soapy water or paraffin oil – a human disposable enema pack also effective.

# CONTAGIOUS EQUINE METRITIS (mare)

This is a highly contagious infection of the uterus caused by a new bacterium isolated in the US, England, France, Ireland and Australia.

SIGNS
Some mares show heavy pus discharge after service – some mares repeatedly come into season after being served.

CAUSE
Bacteria named *Haemophilus equigenitalis.* Mares can be infected by stallion, equipment or personnel.

TREATMENT
Routine swabbing of mares just before stud season – identifies infected mares and symptomless carriers – consult your veterinarian as swabbing technique is complex – set of swabs taken from cervix, clitoral fossa and sinuses at different stages of oestrous cycle. Blood testing for CEM in mares is reliable 19–40 days after infection.

Stud personnel should wear disposable gloves for handling genitalia of mares and stallions – any equipment used should be thoroughy disinfected – use chlorhexidine or similar solution. Bacteria can be treated with range of antibiotics – some mares remain carriers.

# CONTAGIOUS EQUINE METRITIS (stallion)

This is a highly contagious venereal disease, first isolated in England in 1977 and now spread throughout the world. It was identified from mares in Australia late 1977.

SIGNS
Stallions are carriers of contagious equine metritis (CEM) but do not exhibit symptoms – CEM does not cause infertility in stallion – but, by being a carrier, stallion can cause infertility in mare that it serves. The bacteria live in folds and crevices of penis and prepuce. They are transmitted from stallion to stallion if handler touches penis of infected stallion and then touches with his infected hands penis of another stallion – or if equipment used to wash infected stallion's penis after service is used again to wash another stallion's penis.

Finally, CEM can be spread from infected stallion to mare at time of service or by handler touching penis of infected stallion then handling genitals of mare with his contaminated hands. Bacteria also transmitted to stallion when serving an infected mare.

CAUSE
Bacteria (*Haemophilus equigenitalis*).

TREATMENT

Before start of stud season veterinary surgeon should swab penis and prepuce of all stallions and teasers on the stud for bacteriological examination – series of three swabs have to be taken at intervals of not less than 2 days apart before definite diagnosis can be given. CEM highly infectious – all stud personnel should handle external genitalia of mares and stallions wearing disposable gloves – all equipment such as that used to wash stallion's penis should be thoroughly disinfected with chlorhexidine solution after service. It is advisable to consult your veterinary surgeon if there is an infertility problem, as stallion can be treated successfully with complex course of antibiotics.

# CONTRACTED HEELS

SIGNS

Heels close together often with deep furrow between them – frog may be small and hard with shrivelled appearance and not in contact with ground – sole often much more concave than normal – horse may or may not be lame – condition more common in front feet, either one or both.

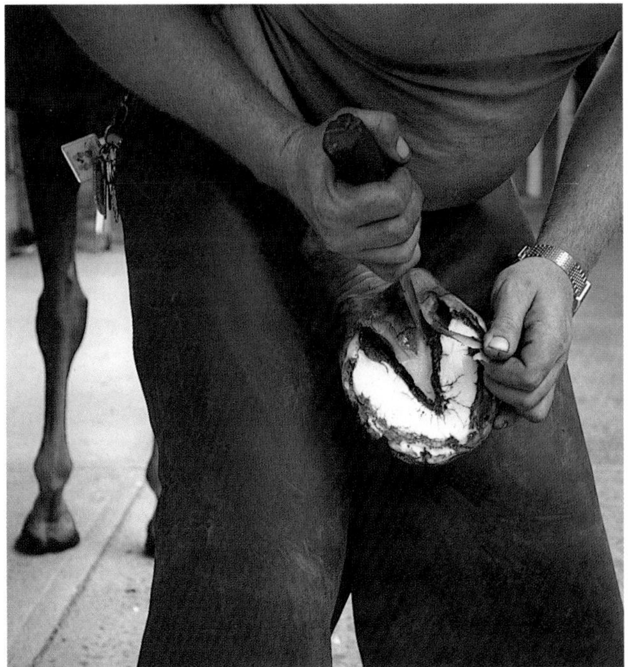

Trimming to lower the heels

CAUSE
Due to frog not being in contact with ground – can be brought about by incorrect trimming and shoeing – or by lameness in the limb – so that when horse moves it does not bring foot, including frog, in proper contact with ground.

TREATMENT
Frog may be made to touch ground by trimming to lower the heels – if not successful a bar shoe can be used to bring pressure to bear on frog, promoting hoof expansion.

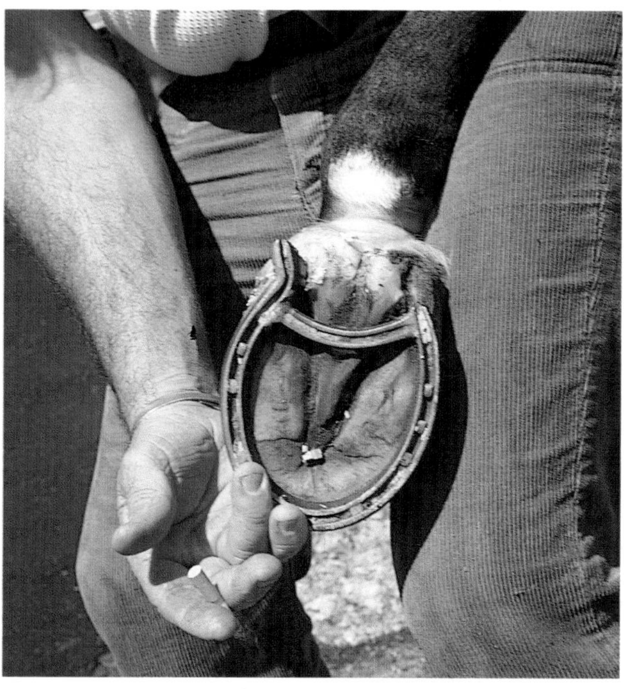

A bar shoe to correct contracted heels

# CONTRACTED TENDONS

SIGNS
Foal stands on its toes or even knuckles over and walks on front of fetlock.

CAUSES
Particular cause of limb deformities difficult to isolate – may be a single one or combination of several – generally, causes may

be classified as nutritional, malpositioning of foal in mare's uterus, inherited genetic abnormalities or injury.

### TREATMENT

Essential to treat deformity as soon as possible to remedy it – failing that, to stabilise it. It is always wise to check nutritional status of mare and foal – if necessary supplement their diet with vitamin and mineral supplement rich in calcium.

Foal should be confined to stable or box to reduce movement to minimum – should be a deep bed of straw to prevent abrasion to skin and to act as cushion and support for legs.

Veterinary surgeon should be called as soon as possible after condition recognised – usual treatment is to apply a brace to back of leg – released about every 2 hours to allow circulation to skin to resume – after 1–2 days brace need no longer be used – in normal cases tendons have stretched to the point where they allow sole of foot to touch ground – once sole of the foot comes in normal contact with ground, movement of foal and weight-bearing effect on tendons will ensure that legs assume normal conformation.

Surgery involving cutting inferior check ligament is a successful procedure – doesn't interfere with normal function of foal's leg.

# CONTUSIONS

### SIGNS

Bruising – swelling of skin and underlying tissue – not necessarily associated with break in skin.

### CAUSES

Kicks – falls – collisions.

### TREATMENT

If no break in skin apply alternately hot and cold foments – make hot foment by putting 2 tablespoons salt in bucket of hot water – just hot enough for your hand to tolerate it – if too hot will scald horse's skin – if lukewarm will not serve purpose of increasing blood circulation – blood aids in skin repair and carrying away damaged tissue. To apply hot foment, soak wad of cotton-wool in bucket of hot water – hold it on contused area till it cools off – do this for 10 minutes – be sure water is kept at same temperature. Follow this procedure by hosing wound area with fair pressure of water for about 5 minutes – repeat hot and cold treatment every 12 hours – hosing water has massaging effect – stimulates circulation and flow of fluid away from site. Danger of infection from any break in skin – guard against with antibiotics.

# CORNEAL ULCER — KERATITIS

Because the cornea, or surface of the eye, is exposed, it is more subject to injury than other parts of the eye. Injury is followed by ulceration. Blindness or poor vision in one or both eyes can make a horse dangerous to ride and ineligible for racing.

Keratitis is inflammation of part or the whole of the cornea. It can occur on its own, following injury or infection, but is also associated with corneal ulcer.

## SIGNS

Tears streaming down cheek – eyelid(s) partially or completely closed – appearance of cornea or surface of affected eye can vary from dull and hazy in a small area to whole corneal surface of eye being opaque and bluish-white in colour – a small pit, varying in depth, may be seen if cornea is ulcerated – scar formation following ulceration is common.

## CAUSES

Dirt or mud may be thrown up from hooves of a horse in front into eyes of horse following – when horses are packed up tightly

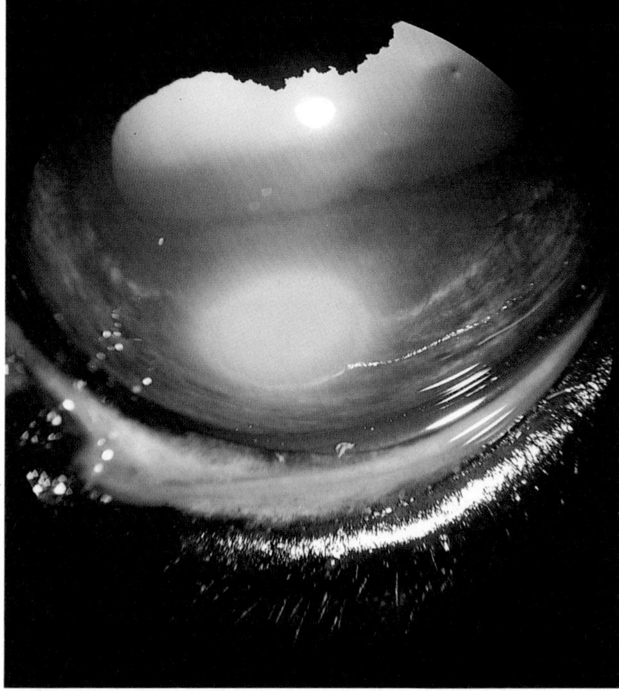

A corneal ulcer highlighted by fluorescent green dye

in race, one may be accidentally hit in eye with a whip – horse being ridden around and between trees and bushes is likely to be poked in eye by a twig – when horse is feeding, a piece of chaff can be blown into the eye – infection can also damage the cornea.

TREATMENT
Call your veterinarian – early treatment will help minimise scar formation and maintain proper vision.

While waiting – bathe eye in hot water and clean it using clean wad of cotton-wool soaked in water of such temperature that your hand can just tolerate the heat – be careful you do not cause further damage to eye while bathing it. Remove horse to shaded area or darken the stable – corneal injury very sensitive to direct sunlight – wind, dust and flies will aggravate problem. If foreign body present and can be readily removed, do so, otherwise leave it for veterinary surgeon to extract.

# CORNS

SIGNS
Collection of blood under sole in region of heel – horse shows signs of lameness.

CAUSE
Commonly caused by heel of shoe turning inwards and putting pressure on sole.

TREATMENT
Correct shoe if necessary – drain blood by carefully paring off minimal amount of sole surface – veterinary surgeon should be called to treat horse with a tetanus injection and antibiotics if infection is present or opened corn is at risk of becoming infected – apply tincture of iodine to opening and cover with adhesive bandage to prevent further contamination – an E–Z boot may also be used.

# CRACKED HEEL

See Greasy Heel (page 216).

# CRIB BITING (Wind Sucking)

SIGNS
Horse grabs solid object with incisor teeth – arches neck – gulps air – can cause gastritis (irritation of stomach) – poor appetite – loss of weight.

CAUSE
Boredom.

TREATMENT
Alleviate boredom by putting hay net in horse box – hen or small goat in horse box as companion – horse out into yard or paddock. Eliminate as many objects as possible that horse can grasp with incisor teeth – commercially available straps placed tightly around neck sometimes effective (see page 295).

# CROSS FIRING

SIGNS
Toe or inside wall of hind foot strikes inside quarter of opposite forefoot – breaks skin, often causing deep wound.

CAUSE
Horses with conformation of toe-out in front feet and toe-in in hind feet – seen in pacers more often than in square trotters or gallopers.

TREATMENT
Toes of forefeet should be rasped square – square-toed shoe fitted – causes forefeet to break in straight line. Hind feet should be fitted with a three-quarter shoe on inside hoof wall to assist hind feet to break in a straight line, preventing interference. Fit horse with bell boots for protection.

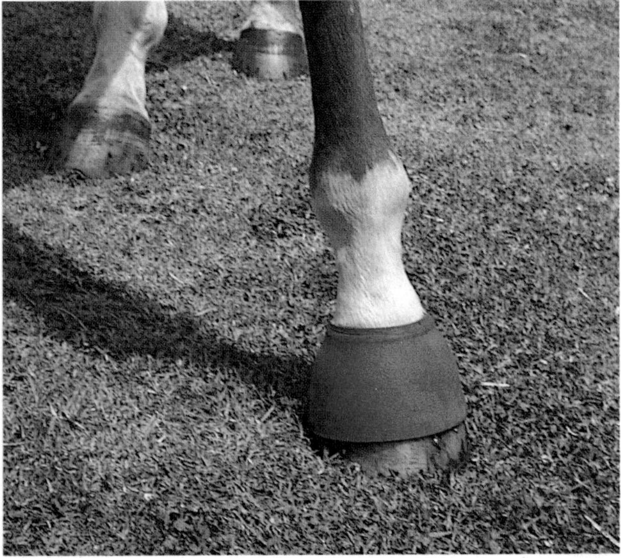

A bell boot

# CURB

Curb is due to the tearing or sprain of a ligament.

SIGNS
Swelling about 10 cm below point of hock – viewed from side is semi-circular in shape – feels hard when pressed – may reduce in size – permanent blemish persists in most cases – horse does not go lame.

CAUSES
Cow or sickle hock conformation – strain from sudden quick movements such as jumping or galloping, especially in muddy conditions – kicking walls, fences and tailgates in floats and trailers.

TREATMENT
Cold hosing – rest – painting twice daily with cooling lotion – all effective treatments. Contact your veterinarian – he may treat condition by administration of anti-inflammatory agent – depending on size of curb. Unless horse has poor conformation, complete recovery usually follows treatment.

# CYSTITIS KIDNEY STONES BLADDER STONES

These diseases are more commonly spoken of as inflammation and infection of the bladder. They are not common in horses; mares are affected more frequently than colts or geldings.

SIGNS
Frequent straining – little or no urine passed – urine may vary in colour – clear to dark red – red a sign of blood being passed – skin around vulva and between legs of mare may be scalded, due to continual dribbling of urine.

CAUSES
Damage to bladder or urethra during foaling – infection of uterus or vagina spreading to bladder – stones in bladder – stones (calculi) usually composed of calcium carbonate – cause of stone formation not clear – may be due to pH (acidity/alkalinity) of urine – infection – or diet (such as certain species of sorghum).

## TREATMENT

Contact your veterinarian – while waiting, collect urine sample in clear glass jar with a screw-top lid – do not use a honey jar – may affect urine sugar level – store sample in refrigerator. If skin scalded by urine – wash area with warm soapy water – dry thoroughly – apply zinc cream or vaseline. Clean, fresh drinking water available to horse at all times. Your veterinarian will administer antibiotics to clear up infection. As preventative – decrease bran and bran feedstuffs in diet – increase water intake by adding 400 g salt daily.

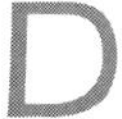

# DEHYDRATION

Horses sweat freely and are often exposed to the environment for lengthy periods in a paddock. Some are regularly and vigorously exercised in preparing for and taking part in such activities as weekend trail riding, racing and endurance riding. They are thus more susceptible than most animals to dehydration, that is, they lose more than normal amounts of fluids and electrolytes that cannot adequately be replenished by normal diet.

Electrolytes are made up of a delicate balance of salts, including sodium, potassium, chloride, bicarbonate, phosphate and magnesium. Body fluids and cells contain electrolyte ions in varying proportions; e.g. body fluids have concentrated sodium and chloride ions, whereas the fluid inside cells contains concentrated potassium ions.

When a cell functions, e.g. when a muscle cell contracts, potassium and other ions from inside the cell pass through the cell wall to the body fluid. Sodium and chloride ions pass from the body fluid to the inside of the muscle cell. Muscle fatigue sets in, i.e. the muscle becomes incapable of further contraction, when the ions in the body fluid equal those within the muscle cell. When the muscles are resting, the reverse action takes place.

Cramping and tying-up result if excessive loss of electrolytes in the sweat is not replaced, because there are insufficient electrolytes in the horse's diet to restore the correct balance. Daily feeding of an electrolyte mixture will ensure that electrolytes are replaced as they are lost and this will prevent dehydration. There is a limit to the quantity of electrolytes a horse will accept in its feed. Horses in training or performance horses that require greater amounts of electrolytes can be given them by stomach tube.

## SIGNS

Dry harsh coat – sunken eyes – lethargy – loss of appetite – hard, dry balls of manure – fatigue – cramping – tying-up – lack of will to win – poor performance and poor recovery from exercise – when skin pinched, lack of return or slow return to normal.

## CAUSE

Continual loss of electrolytes and fluid through faeces (droppings), sweat and urine – accelerated by the following factors –

exercise, heat, travelling, diarrhoea, loss of appetite, lack of access to water and free sweating.

TREATMENT
Balanced electrolyte mixture can be administered orally by means of feed or drinking water – by nasal stomach tube (electrolytes being dissolved in water) – intravenously (electrolytes being contained in specially prepared sterile solution).

Blood tests can be done to evaluate which electrolyte is deficient – solution concentrated in deficient electrolyte can then be administered. Drugs that act on the kidney can be injected into horse, causing retention of certain ions in the body.

# DENTAL CAPS

SIGNS
Slow eating – excessive salivation – quidding food (i.e. dropping partially chewed food from mouth) – masticating food difficult.

CAUSE
Head or crown of permanent molar becomes locked into roots of temporary molar as permanent molar is erupting through gum – remains of temporary molar attached to head of permanent molar is known as a dental cap.

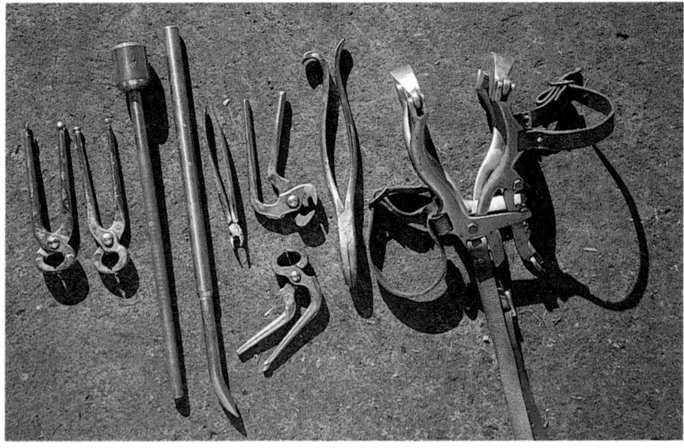

Equipment for teeth care

TREATMENT
Remove cap with tooth forceps or lever off cap by inserting suitable instrument, e.g. screwdriver, between cap and permanent tooth.

# DEPRAVED APPETITE

Eating manure, bedding and dirt is an unpleasant, unhealthy habit sometimes acquired by horses.

SIGNS
Horse eating dung – suspicion aroused when mucking out stable or yard – little or no dung found – keep in mind horse may be constipated.

CAUSES
Poor nutrition – vitamin and mineral deficiencies – boredom in being confined to small yard – stable – insufficient food – lack of access to natural grazing pasture. Presence of sweet additives in feed – honey – glucose – molasses – powdered milk – give dung sweet taste.

TREATMENT
Provide well-balanced mineral and vitamin supplement – adequate quantities of good quality feed – remove sweet additives from diet. Relieve boredom by giving horse access to paddock with good quality pasture – if not available provide hay net with good quality lucerne hay. Remove dung from stable or yard four times daily. Regular worming program essential.

# DIARRHOEA

This condition may also be referred to as scouring, and some cases are difficult to treat. If unchecked in the first 2 days of a foal's life, it often results in death. It is uncommon in mature horses. Many cases can be prevented by proper management: feeding, worming, teeth care and cleanliness. Call the veterinarian immediately – once the causative organism is identified appropriate drugs can be administered.

SIGNS
Disease recognised if dung is cow-like, or like porridge or discoloured fluid – horse with diarrhoea usually recognised by state of its tail and hindquarters – shows signs of discomfort when passing motion – switching tail – looking at flank – tucking up abdomen. Colour of faeces may vary – pale to yellow to black with streaks of blood and mucus. Horse's appetite fluctuates from normal to non-existent. If diarrhoea severe – may show signs of colic. If diarrhoea continues – horse loses weight – becomes weak – depressed – dehydrated.

CAUSES
Bad teeth – broken teeth – teeth with sharp edges – all lead to incomplete mastication. Quantity and quality of food – too much

succulent lucerne or clover or mouldy hay. Other causes may be bacterial – viral – protozoal – excitement – nervousness.

TREATMENT
Call your veterinarian – will treat symptoms and try to find cause – treatment for diarrhoea caused by worms entirely different from treatment for diarrhoea caused by salmonella. Things you can do – isolate horse – reduce its volume of feed by half or give it none at all – remove from its diet succulent lucerne and hay, bran, powdered milk – replace with oaten hay – give horse frequent small amounts of water with electrolytes – check teeth and date of last worming – assess quality of feed recently given to horse – reduce its exercise – move to another paddock, out of sight, if disturbed by other horses. If horse doesn't respond turn out for lengthy spell.

# DIARRHOEA (foal)

SIGNS
Temperature rise – colic may be present – motion fluid and putrid – lethargy – lacks appetite – if unchecked, possible death, particularly in first two days of life.

CAUSES
Foal greedy drinker and mare good milk supplier – restrict foal's milk intake by milking mare – milk intake for foal should be a little, often. Foal ingests mare's faeces – diarrhoea often results – immediately remove mare's droppings – best form of control. Mare comes on heat 9–12 days after foaling – heat period lasts 3–5 days – during this period foal may have diarrhoea – condition ends when mare goes off heat.

TREATMENT
Call veterinarian – provide good nursing – keep foal warm and protected from elements – provide clean water and electrolytes – isolate foal from others – disinfect stable or box in which foal housed – decrease foal's milk and water intake – frequently remove dung from stable.

# DOURINE

Dourine is encountered mainly in the tropics and sub-tropical areas.

SIGNS
*Early stage:* swelling of penis and prepuce – scrotum and testicles become swollen – genitalia of mare and stallion covered with blisters, pustules and ulcers.

*Later stage:* weakness of hindquarters – knuckling – stumbling – circular swellings of skin 2–4 cm in size on croup, shoulder, chest and abdomen – appear and disappear rapidly – persistent lesions of head and external genitalia become hard and lose their pigment.
*Terminal cases:* hypersensitive to touch – ticklishness and paralysis of hindquarters – severe weight loss – stallion lies down.

## CAUSE

Infection by *Trypanosoma equiperdum* is spread at time of service or by use of contaminated equipment. Biting insects may be involved in transmission.

## TREATMENT

Your veterinarian will make definite diagnosis by pathological examination of blood and secretions – disease should be suspected if number of mares develop characteristic genital lesions when served by same stallion. Veterinarian can treat both stallion and mare with specific drugs. Stallion and mare should not be used for breeding – stallion should be castrated.

# E

## EAR MITES

The presence of ear mites is not common. Sometimes the signs are not obvious to the unpractised eye and the problem goes undetected for a long time.

SIGNS
One or both ears tend to droop – horse very sensitive to ears being touched or putting on bridle – rubbing ears – shaking head – holding head on one side – dark wax discharge from ear.

CAUSE
Presence in ears of tiny mites.

TREATMENT
Contact your veterinarian – will examine wax from ear canal under microscope – mites in the wax give positive diagnosis – veterinarian will then prescribe correct ear drops. A twitch and/or tranquilliser may have to be used so that ears can be thoroughly cleaned of all wax and prescribed drops applied.

## ENTROPION

Entropion is a turning in of the eyelid, causing the eyelashes to rub on the surface of the eyeball (cornea) and irritate it.

SIGNS
Weeping of affected eye – evidenced by continual wet patch below it – partial closure of eyelid of affected eye or rubbing eye to alleviate constant irritation – closer examination reveals upper and/or lower eyelid turned in, causing eyelashes to rub on surface of eyeball, thus irritating it.

CAUSES
Some foals born with condition – often both eyes affected – lower eyelid more commonly involved. Chronic conjunctivitis and lacerations of eyelids can cause entropion in adult horses.

TREATMENT

Contact your veterinarian – condition can be successfully cured by surgery – in young foals the affected lid may be corrected by turning out lid six or more times a day and applying an eye ointment.

# EPIPHYSITIS

Most well-muscled, well-grown yearlings and 2-year-olds are skeletally immature. You may have a horse in which the flesh (muscle) is willing but the skeleton (bone and associated ligaments, tendons and connective tissue) is weak. Many horses are not skeletally mature until they are about 4½ years old.

Many yearlings and 2-year-olds have open epiphyseal lines that cannot be seen by looking at the knees (these are not related to the term 'open knees'). A long bone during its growth possesses a long middle part, known as the shaft or diaphysis, and two ends, each known as an epiphysis. During development the epiphysis is not fused with the diaphysis but is actually separated from it by the epiphyseal line. In the growing stage this line is said to be open; at maturity the epiphyses fuse with the diaphysis and the epiphyseal line disappears, and is said to be closed. The only way to evaluate the epiphyseal line is by X-ray.

Areas normally evaluated by the veterinarian are knees and hocks as the epiphyseal lines in these areas are the last to close. X-rays taken approximately 2.5 cm above the knee will reveal the extent of the epiphyseal line closure. The degree of closure of the epiphyseal line indicates the general maturity or immaturity of the whole skeleton, as well as the degree of development in the local area.

Horses with closed epiphyseal lines are usually ready to be broken in, educated and worked. Those with partially closed epiphyseal lines may be broken in then spelled to allow maturation to take place. Horses with open epiphyseal lines should be spelled, otherwise the stress of breaking-in and education could cause epiphysitis, shin soreness, splints, fractures, poor development or chronic lameness, all leading to unsoundness.

There are normal closure times for each epiphyseal line which vary with different breeds of horses, nutritional levels and certain diseases.

SIGNS

Swelling 2.5 cm above knee – seen in yearlings and 2-year-olds when being broken in (educated) or trained – pain may be evident on palpation of swelling or flexion of knee – if lame, there is stilted, proppy action in affected leg.

### CAUSES
Educating, working immature horses – feeding high-grain diets high in phosphorus and low in calcium.

### TREATMENT
Blood count should be taken to evaluate calcium and phosphorus levels – diet can be adjusted to correct any imbalance that may adversely affect epiphyseal closure. Horses with open epiphyseal lines on X-ray should be spelled. Anabolic steroids may be used in selected cases with beneficial effect – they help the process of epiphyseal closure and speed up the maturation of the yearling's skeleton.

# EQUINE INFECTIOUS ANAEMIA

This is a viral infection of horses which occurs worldwide.

### SIGNS
Incubation period 8–14 days – varies according to whether disease is acute or chronic.
*Acute:* temperature over 40°C – weakness – wobbly – muscle tremor – yellow, inflamed mucous membranes – fluid swelling (oedema) under belly and in legs – exercise produces pounding heartbeat – anaemia develops later – usually continues eating – death may occur.
*Chronic:* weight loss – poor performance – exhaustion – severe anaemia – horse may recover with attacks occurring less frequently – or can die unexpectedly in acute relapse. Horses that apparently recover remain carriers of virus.

### CAUSES
Virus transmitted by biting insects (horse flies, biting midges) – by use of non-sterile needles and blood-contaminated surgical instruments.

### TREATMENT
Disease diagnosed by pathology test (Coggins Test) – no specific treatment – good nursing – rest – high protein feed – antibiotics for treatment of secondary infection. Many countries require negative Coggins Test before horse allowed in.

# EQUINE INFLUENZA

In mid-1950s, horses in Sweden were diagnosed as having a respiratory infection caused by an influenza virus. In 1957, a closely related virus infected horses in the US and again, in 1963, a new strain of influenza virus affected most horses there. The disease is widespread in France, England and Ireland.

## SIGNS

Readily observed sign is dry cough, persisting sometimes for 3 weeks. Initially, nasal discharge is clear and watery, progressing to thick mucus. A high temperature over 4-day period often indicates developing pneumonia. Loss of appetite – lethargy – generalised muscular weakness are consistent with viral infections. Foals and older horses or horses under stress, such as those in work or being transported, are more susceptible to viruses and secondary bacterial infections.

## CAUSE

Two strains of equine influenza virus can live for up to 2 days in nasal mucus – provided environmental conditions suitable. Virus destroyed by heat, light, formalin, soaps and detergents.

Respiratory viruses are spread by horses coughing droplets of infected mucus – then inhaled by healthy horse. By having heavy mucus running from nose, horses may contaminate pasture – healthy horse inhales virus as it grazes – a group of horses will develop same symptoms in 1–3 days because of highly contagious nature of these viruses.

## TREATMENT

Rest from work for 3 weeks is important to allow mucous membrane lining of respiratory tract to heal. Protect horse from environment – rug and stable it from the cold and wind – provide shade in very hot weather. Make water available at all times and provide high-quality, nutritious diet.

Contact your veterinarian – if secondary bacterial infection evident – will administer course of antibiotics and treat horse according to its symptoms. Isolate the horse from others. Overcrowding should be avoided. In US, England, Ireland and Europe, vaccine is available that offers immunity only if a series of injections are given. Disinfect stables, feed bins and water buckets if contaminated.

# EQUINE VIRAL ARTERITIS

SIGNS

Pregnant mares may abort during illness or shortly after – incubation period of 2–6 days – horse's symptoms may be high temperature (42°C) – off food – dopey – weak – inflamed discoloured eyes – nasal discharge. Some show oedema (swelling) in legs, udder and underbelly – constipation – colic – diarrhoea.

CAUSE

Virus worldwide but not in Australia – transmitted by direct contact – droplets from sneezing, coughing, eating – nasal discharge – saliva.

TREATMENT

Rest for 1 month after signs disappear – alter diet – if constipated, feed bran mash – if diarrhoea, dry feed – isolate infected horses, stalls and grazing area – disinfect stable area – contact your veterinarian for antibiotics – eye ointment – electrolytes and fluids – good immunity persists after natural infection.

# EQUINE VIRAL RHINOPNEUMONITIS

SIGNS

Incubation period of infection about 2 weeks – symptoms of a cold – temperature up – nasal discharge – coughing – sneezing – respiratory disease – abortion may occur up to 4 months after infection when mare appears healthy – abortion usually occurs from 5th month onwards. Foetus expelled rapidly with placenta – virus can affect brain and spinal cord of mare causing paralysis of the hindquarters – foetus aborted after 6 months shows discolouration of placental fluid and hooves due to diarrhoea in uterus. Disease found throughout world including Australia.

CAUSE

Virus enters horse through respiratory tract – in the young and weak causes bronchitis and pneumonia – some cases carry the virus without symptoms – virus spread by direct contact – droplets from sneezing, coughing, feeding, drinking – contact with aborted foetus or its membrane – if group of pregnant mares infected with virus you have abortion epidemic.

TREATMENT

None specific – antibiotics – rest – isolate new mares for 3 weeks – isolate aborted mares – burn or bury aborted material – disinfect stalls and abortion area with Formalin – keep weanlings some distance from brood mares – vaccination in US and UK – contact your veterinarian.

# F

## FISTULOUS WITHERS

Fistulas are long, pipe-like, narrow-mouthed ulcers that may appear on the withers as non-infected, localised swellings or as an extensive weeping infection, starting at the withers and running under the skin, sometimes along two-thirds of the shoulder blade. To prevent the formation of fistulas, check that the saddle fits the withers properly. Correct saddling procedure should be followed as a matter of routine.

### SIGNS

Disease may erupt suddenly with all signs of acute inflammation such as swelling, heat and pain – it may develop slowly and insidiously without any obvious signs of inflammation, the first real sign being discharge at point of eruption. Fistulas may develop on one or both sides of withers – horse stiff in movements of forelimbs.

When swelling erupts – fluid is straw-coloured – in few days changes to whitish-yellow discharge of pus. Site of eruption may dry up – heal and scar – later another eruption will occur in different spot on withers.

### CAUSES

Infection – bacteria found in discharge are same as those that cause abortion in cattle and poll evil in horses. Trauma – in most cases injury to withers by saddle precedes infection. In few cases no observable evidence that trauma or infection is cause.

### TREATMENT

If small, localised swelling develops on or near withers, do not use a saddle on horse until swelling has disappeared completely and skin has regained its toughness and elasticity. If horse in training, its fitness program can be continued by lungeing, leading off a pony and swimming.

Bathe swelling 4 times a day for 10 minutes each time, using water just hot enough for hand to tolerate – apply a drawing agent such as Magnoplasm or antiphlogistine.

If infected area extensive, involving sinuses running under skin, surgical drainage as well as administration of antibiotics is necessary. Call your veterinarian – he will take swab from discharge to identify bacteria and determine what antibiotic is most effective – a lengthy course of antibiotics is administered at a high level because condition likely to recur.

Place water and feed containers at appropriate height when horse is suffering from fistulas – some horses refuse to bend down because of pain.

# FLY AND MOSQUITO BITES

Stable flies and mosquitoes can cause an allergic-type skin reaction. If the horse is rugged, numerous small nodules are found in the areas where the skin is exposed.

## SIGNS

House fly seems to be attracted to corners of horse's eyes – causes conjunctivitis and weeping – in turn attracts more flies – stable fly is larger than house fly – has savage bite – can attack horse on any part of body – most attracted to legs – when attacked horse becomes restless, stamps its feet, switches its tail and bites skin where bitten if it can reach it – raised lumps, up to 1 cm in diameter, often appear at site of fly bite.

## CAUSE

House fly and stable fly commonly cause irritation – both are prolific breeders in soiled bedding and manure.

## TREATMENT

Similar to treatment for conjunctivitis – use of fly veils and fly-repellent ointment applied around eyes helpful – if possible put horse in stable with fly screens on windows and doors – rug it with fly sheet.

Fly spray and pest strips in stable help to reduce fly population – spraying horse with pyrethrum effective for several hours – frequent removal of soiled bedding and manure to flyproof manure storage pit also a preventive measure in control of flies.

# FOAL PNEUMONIA (Rattles)

Rattles is the common name for pneumonia because of the rattling sound in the chest that accompanies breathing. It is an infectious disease of young foals, occurring in most countries. The problem appears to localise itself to certain studs in any one area, suggesting that it may be due to management.

## SIGNS

Coughing, especially when moving, and a loud noise (rattles) due to moisture in lungs – accompanied by laboured breathing, often stimulated by handling – foal has harsh coat – an elevated temperature.

CAUSE
Bacterium known as *Corynebacterium equi* is causative agent – can enter foal's body via stump of umbilical cord, via placenta while the foal is in uterus or via migrating roundworm larvae. In some cases it is unknown how bacteria enter living tissue of the foal.

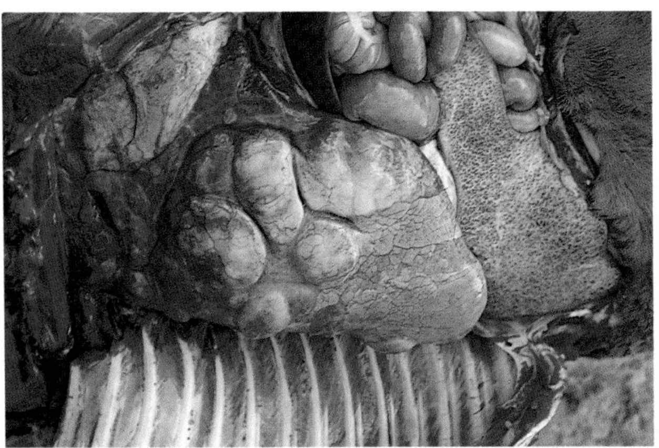

Rattles: abscesses in the lung tissue seen during post-mortem

TREATMENT
Call veterinary surgeon – in meantime keep foal confined, warm and well-nourished.

Rattles can be controlled: establish a program of priorities – such as a routine of giving antibiotics at birth if disease is common on stud – isolate infected foals – clean yards and boxes regularly – establish a well-organised worming procedure – maintain a good nutrition program.

# FOALING

As an owner, you may be distressed or disturbed witnessing a birth, especially by the mare's strenuous labour and the afterbirth dangling from the vulva, but remember it is normal. Inform your veterinarian about two weeks before the approximate time of birth.

## SIGNS

All signs not always present. Pre-birth signs may be mare large and swollen – wants to be alone – muscle shrinkage both sides of croup – bagging up of udder – wax-like secretion from teats. Imminent birth signs may be mare restless – agitated – sweating – pawing ground – stretching – swishing tail – lying down, getting up – fluid from vagina (not to be mistaken for urine) – straining – foetal membrane appears at vagina – may have been ruptured by foal's feet.

## TREATMENT

Provide suitable bedding for labour – grassy spot – deep clean straw bedding in a sterile box or stable 3.5 metres square. Have equipment at hand for birth – iodine – cotton-wool – towelling – 2 buckets for hot water – disinfectant – Hibiclens – surgical gloves – lubricant. As head of foal appears – remove any foetal membrane obstructing nostrils. Umbilical cord as a rule breaks naturally about 5–8 cm from navel, maybe when foal struggles to its feet or when mare rises – swab cord stump with iodine – in 2–3 weeks it will wither – drop off – leave neat navel.

Within 3 hours after foaling – mare expels placental membrane (afterbirth) – normal for it to hang from mare's vulva for up to about 8 hours – never remove it by force – spread out afterbirth on ground to check its complete removal – if you think mare has not expelled it all – call your veterinarian. When foaling finished – cleanse mare – check for tears, bruising, swelling, vaginal discharge, udder infection and inverted nipples.

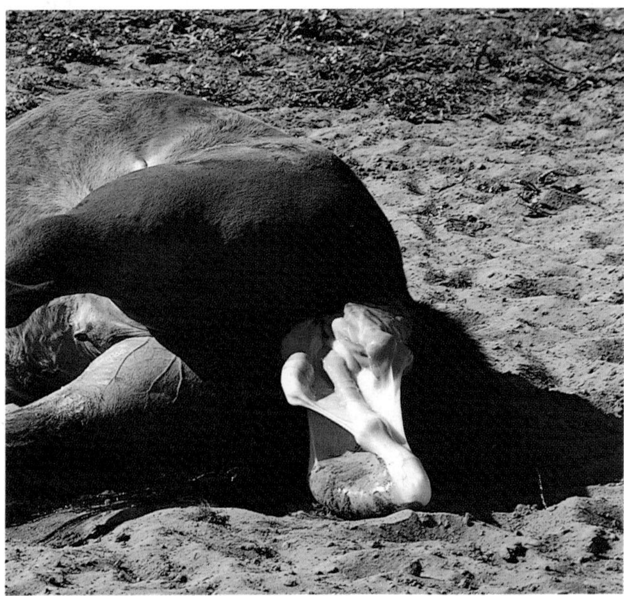

The foal's front feet appear at the vulva in the amnion

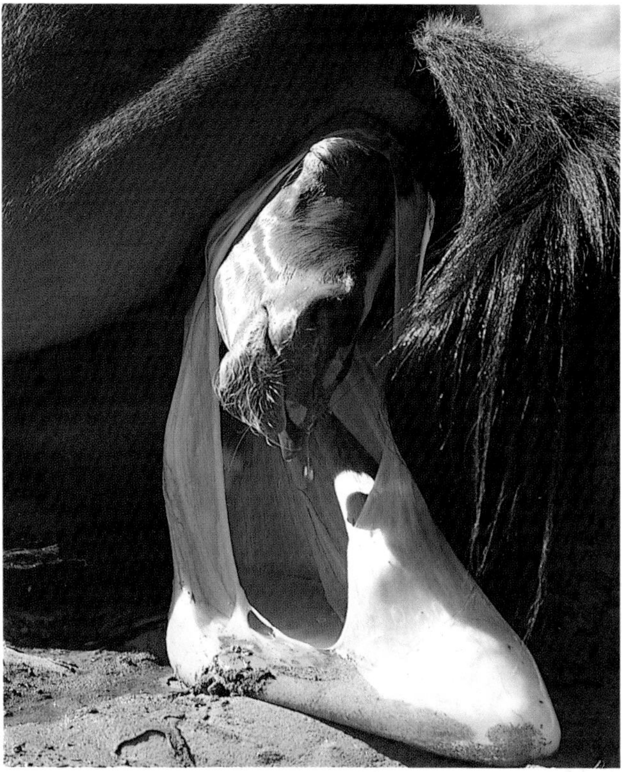

The head, resting on the forelegs, appears through the vulva

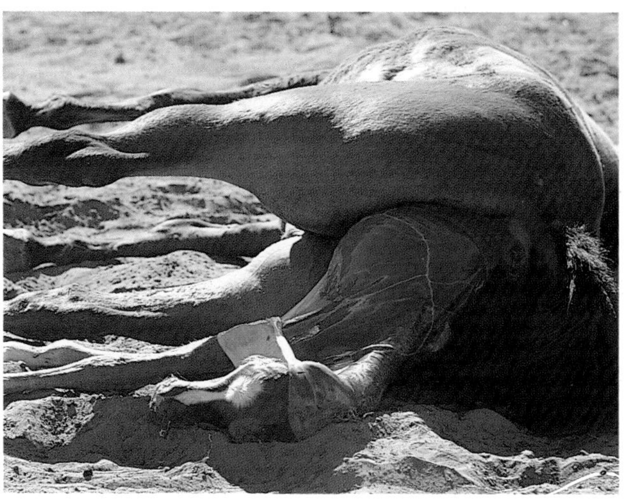

The head is followed by shoulders and chest

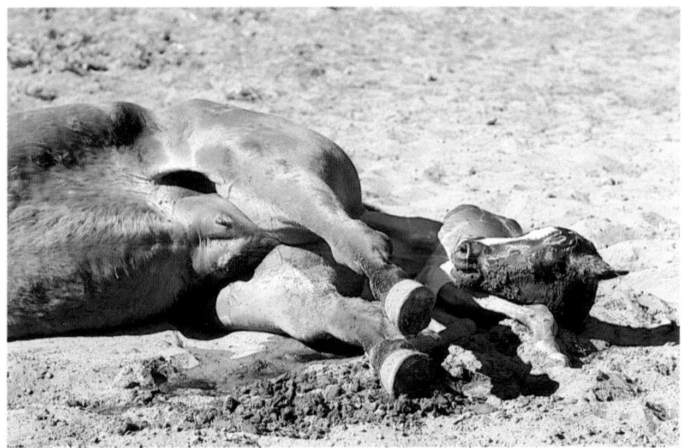

The birth is over — mare and foal take a well-earned rest

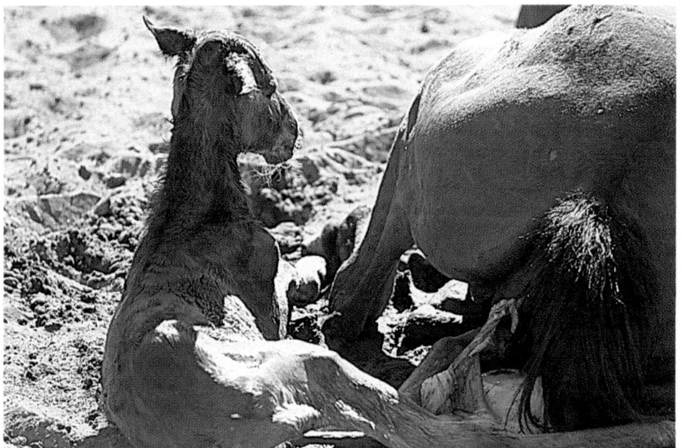

The umbilical cord is intact when the foal is born

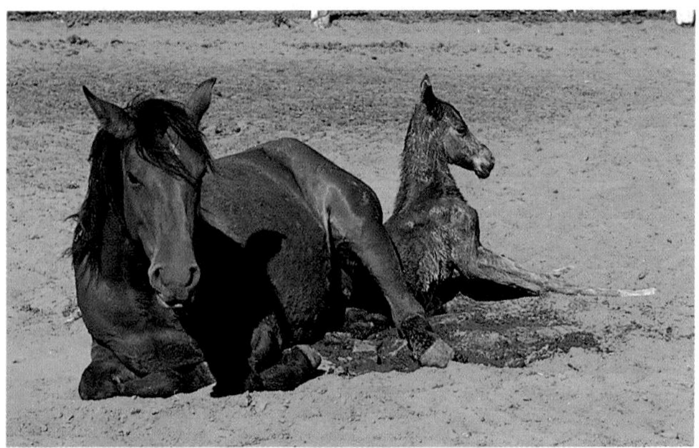

The foal makes awkward movements to get to its feet

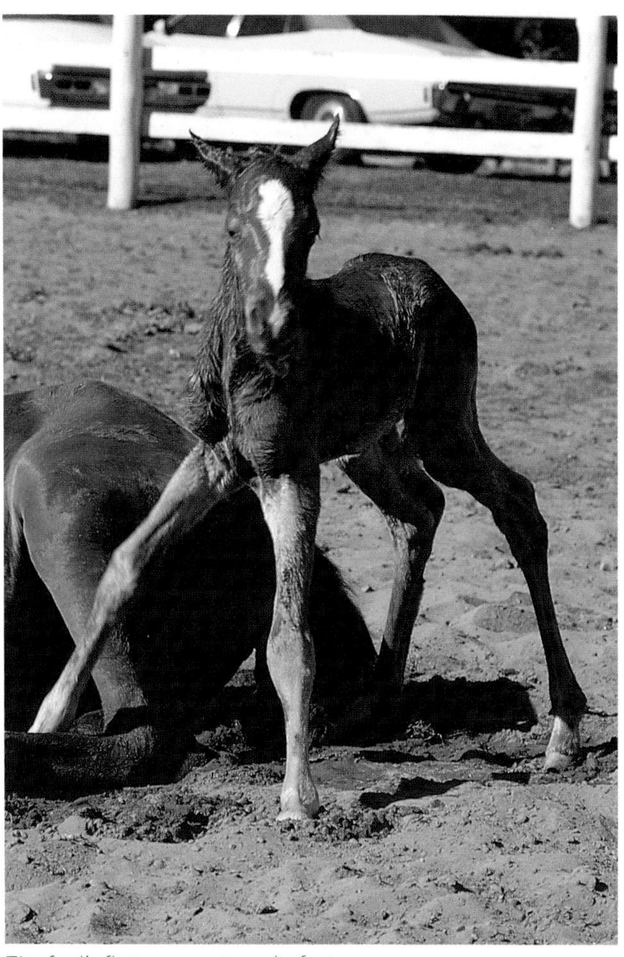

The foal's first moments on its feet

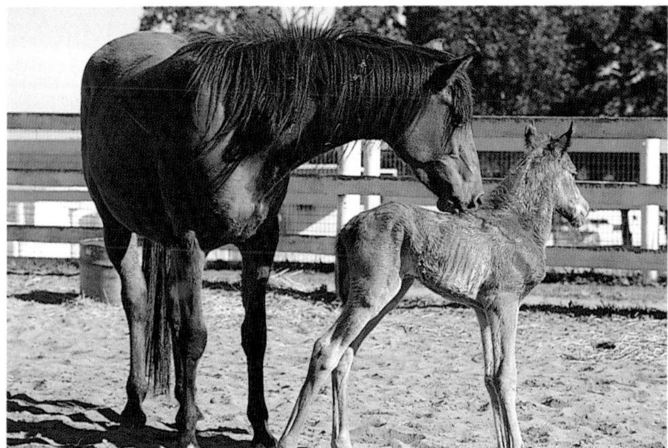

The mare is on her feet, nuzzling and licking the foal

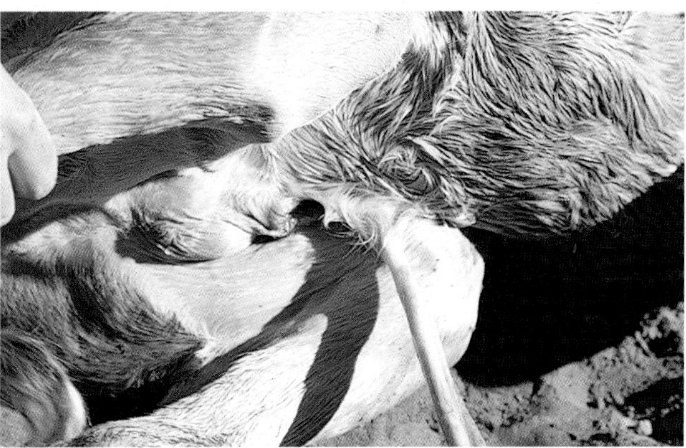

An unbroken umbilical cord

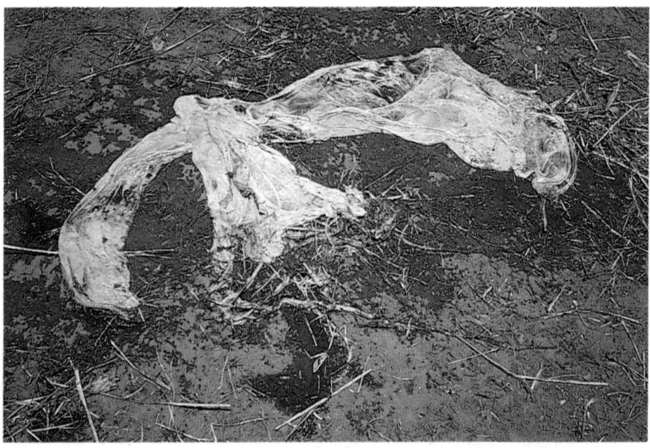

Examine the afterbirth to check it has all been expelled

# FOUNDER (Laminitis)

'Founder' and 'laminitis' are synonymous; both terms are used to describe inflammation of the sensitive laminae that cover the pedal bone inside the hoof. The condition can be acute or chronic. It is usually confined to the front feet though all four feet may be involved.

SIGNS

Horse reluctant to move – tends to lie down or change its weight continually from one foot to another – if only front feet involved horse will stand with hind legs well up under body and its forelegs well forward – this position adopted so that as much weight as possible is taken off front feet – if forced to move horse will shuffle along, putting heels to ground first – affected feet are hot due to inflammation and increased arterial blood supply – throbbing of arteries running down either side of pastern can be felt with slight pressure of fingers.

Horse refuses to eat, sweats and trembles – symptoms reflect pain that horse is suffering – in severe cases its hoof or hooves may fall off – with chronic cases, horse is intermittently lame, putting heels of affected feet to ground first – feet are often warm – sole dropped and convex instead of being concave – ring-like impressions are present on hoof wall.

CAUSES

Ingestion of excessive amounts of grain, particularly wheat and barley – drinking large amounts of water while still hot after exercise – ingestion of excessive amount of lush pasture – intermittent, severe exercise on hard surfaces. Other causes are retention of placenta after foaling, diarrhoea and other gut disorders. Some causes unknown.

TREATMENT

If horse has acute founder, contact your veterinary surgeon – while waiting for him to examine and treat horse, you can help by removing cause if possible – e.g. if horse has been eating an excessive amount of grain, change it to grain-free diet.

You may cool horse's feet in a variety of ways – by hosing them – by packing them in ice – by standing horse in a dam, stream or wet muddy area – if not available naturally, create it. It is a good idea to move horse about for short periods at frequent intervals to stimulate circulation in feet. Feed horse with warm bran mash as a gentle laxative (see page 45).

Some horses recover completely from acute founder – depends on its cause, severity and speed of treatment. If rotation of third phalanx (pedal bone) has taken place, chance of recovery not good.

Treatment for chronic founder is long-term – covers use of anti-inflammatory agents prescribed by your veterinary surgeon.

It also involves corrective trimming and shoeing – heels are trimmed and rasped as much as possible with minimal or no rasping of ground surface of wall at the toe. A wide bar shoe is placed on foot to protect it and to prevent further dropping of sole, caused by downward rotation of pedal bone. In some cases, corrective trimming and shoeing over long period of time can slowly but surely restore foot to original state.

# FRACTURE

Until recently, if a horse broke its leg it was destroyed. With today's advanced surgical, medical and engineering techniques, this is not the case. Most fractures encountered in the horse involve bones of limbs.

SIGNS
One or more of following signs may be evident: lameness – swelling – pain – haemorrhage – anxiety – sweating – trembling – limb hanging limply or bone protruding.

CAUSE
Fractures in many cases due to repeated concussion or to synchronisation failure between joint and muscles that operate it – forelimbs are more susceptible to concussion than hind ones

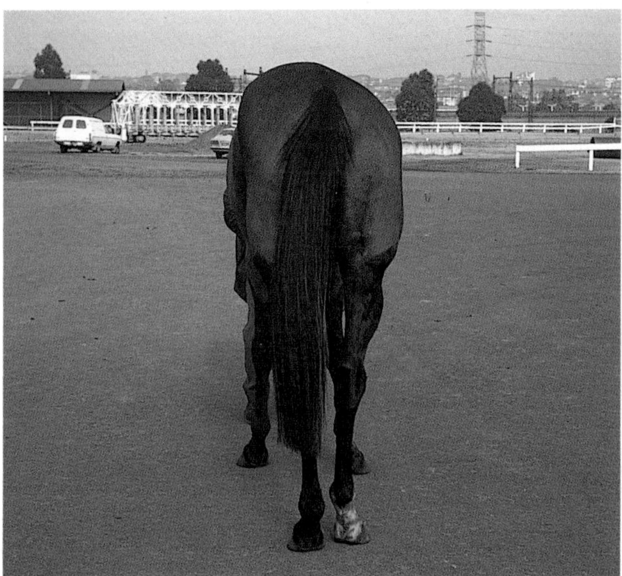

Fractured hip: the rump is lopsided

as latter are protected by constant flexion of joints of limb, particularly stifle and hock – forelimb from elbow down is completely locked into a rigid rod when horse is standing squarely on all four feet – horse in motion bears far greater weight on forelimbs than on hind limbs – forelimbs are therefore subject to more fractures and injuries from concussion and trauma than rear limbs – not only do they bear weight of body in movement but also aid hind limbs in propelling it forward.

## TREATMENT

If horse has obvious fracture of lower limb, apply a splint to prevent any further damage at site of fracture while waiting for veterinarian – splint can be readily made by wrapping pillow or roll of cotton-wool around leg with its centre over fracture – bind pillow or cotton-wool to leg with crepe bandages applied as tightly as possible – to add extra rigidity, a broom handle is incorporated in bandage, with a final few layers of 75 mm Elastoplast applied as tightly as possible – splint not only immobilises fracture – also helps relieve certain amount of pain.

Many factors influence prognosis for healing of fractures – immature horses are more likely to recover from fractures than adults – lighter, smaller horses have a better chance of fracture healing than larger breeds – a quiet, docile temperament is also important – fractures of bones that bear weight directly have a

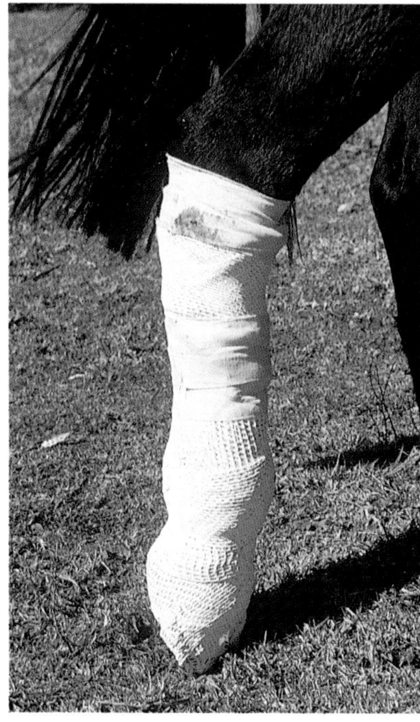

Fractured leg in a fibreglass cast

poorer prognosis than fractures of bones that do not – fractures of lower limb usually have better chance of healing than those above knee and hock – compound and commuted fractures have reduced chances of successful repair.

Fractures can vary from small chip fracture of knee – size of thumb nail – to a completely shattered humerus or femur.

Repair is brought about by what is called closed reduction or open reduction. Closed reduction is technique used to immobilise a fracture with material such as splints, fibreglass and plaster casts. Open reduction involves surgery, when an incision is made and ends of fractured bone are immobilised by use of pins, plates, screws and wire – metal used for these is of an inert nature so that surrounding tissues do not reject device – radiographs are taken to determine what method of reduction is to be used and what type of immobilisation is to be employed.

Immobilisation of fractures in horse poses problem of finding materials strong and rigid enough to combat weight and strength of horse, as well as allowing it to remain mobile. Today, with improvement in production of plaster and fibreglass, casts can be applied to a horse's leg under general anaesthetic that dry and develop great strength and rigidity before horse starts to move about when recovering from anaesthetic.

For certain fractures, such as those of sesamoid bones, splint bones, and chip fractures in the knee, surgical removal of fragments is best treatment.

A recent development in treatment of major fractures of legs is immersion tank – horse, with fractured leg immobilised, is placed in tank containing saline solution – its buoyant effect provides support and immobilisation during healing.

# G

## GENETIC PROBLEMS (stallion)

SIGNS
Small testicles – hard on palpation – may be fairly inactive – poor quality semen – lack of libido. Horse may have testicles that have failed to descend (cryptorchidism) – cannot be used as a stallion – sterile. The monorchid is horse with only one testicle descended (called a rig). Hernias – umbilical and inguinal (groin) – may be result of inherited predisposition.

CAUSE
Genetic defect.

TREATMENT
Though monorchid is fertile, should not be used as stallion because condition thought to be hereditary. This recommendation would still apply even if other testicle, through use of hormones, could be made to descend and develop.

Hernias could mechanically hinder stallion serving or cause pain when mounting – also risk of loop of intestine strangulating in hernial ring.

## GETTING DOWN BEHIND

SIGNS
When cantering or galloping, back or fetlock of hind limbs touches ground, grazing skin, sometimes severely.

CAUSE
Horses with long sloping pasterns are more prone to this problem, as are horses with a foot with long toe and low heel.

TREATMENT
Toe of foot of offending leg should be cut back as short as possible – leave heel intact – horse can be shod with a variety of shoes, depending on severity of problem – shoe with extended heel, with raised heel, or a bar shoe should suffice – bandaging helps to protect skin.

# GLANDERS

Glanders has been eliminated in most well-developed countries, although it is still prevalent as a contagious disease in some of the less-developed parts of the world. Man is susceptible to the disease and in some cases it is fatal.

SIGNS
Horses that develop chronic form of the disease show weight loss – nasal discharge – coughing – pneumonia – ulcerations of nasal cavity and of skin erupting on inside of hock – nodules under skin are up to 2 cm in diameter – discharge a honey-like pus.

CAUSE
Bacterium *Actinobacillus mallei* is causative agent – survives in water for up to 4 weeks – readily destroyed by desiccation from sun and by certain disinfectants such as iodine – infection mainly by ingestion – may be by inhalation or by abrasion of skin.

TREATMENT
Isolate horse(s) – contact your veterinary surgeon or appropriate authority immediately.

# GREASY HEEL

This is a dermatitis or inflammation of the skin at the back of the pastern and between the heels. It is found more frequently in the hind limbs than the forelimbs.

SIGNS
Affected areas sore to touch. In early stages, skin inflamed, after which it becomes raw and bleeds – hair loss and deep cracks with thickened skin on either side may develop. In severe cases, swelling of pastern and fetlock accompany lameness.

CAUSES
Standing or exercising in wet or muddy conditions predisposes skin to infection – skin at back of pastern may be abraded by exercising on sandy surfaces or by rope burns – if area constantly wet and washed with soap it may become irritated.

TREATMENT
Keep horse's legs as dry as possible – reduce hosing to minimum – put horse in well-drained, dry yard – work it on dry surfaces – wipe any grit from backs of pasterns and from between

heels after exercise – grit can have an abrasive action, especially when embedded in cracks in skin.

If skin condition old, dry and hard, apply zinc cream to soften skin and minimise cracking – if skin moist and oozing, apply gentian violet to dry it out – leave skin open to air – bandages often keep surface moist and collect grit that acts like sandpaper – if pasterns swollen and oozing, call your veterinary surgeon for professional advice and treatment.

# GUTTURAL POUCH, INFECTED (contains pus)

# GUTTURAL POUCH – TYMPANY (contains trapped air)

The Eustachian tube extends for about 10 cm from the middle ear to the throat. A section of it is distended to form a sac known as the guttural pouch. These pouches are found only in horses and other solipeds; their precise function is obscure.

SIGNS

Swelling below ear, on one or both sides – where head meets neck – discomfort – breathing difficult. When tapped with fingers swelling may be firm, containing pus, or make hollow sound indicating it contains air. Discharge from one or both nostrils depending on whether one or both guttural pouches are involved – often nasal discharge obvious when horse puts head to ground.

TREATMENT

Surgery recommended. Call your veterinarian.

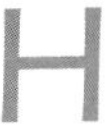

# HAEMATOMA

This is a circumscribed swelling of variable size and position, located under the skin and containing blood.

SIGNS

Generally occurs in area of muscle masses – size varies up to that of a football – usually not sore to touch – in early stage soft to touch – when tapped feels like fluid-filled cavity.

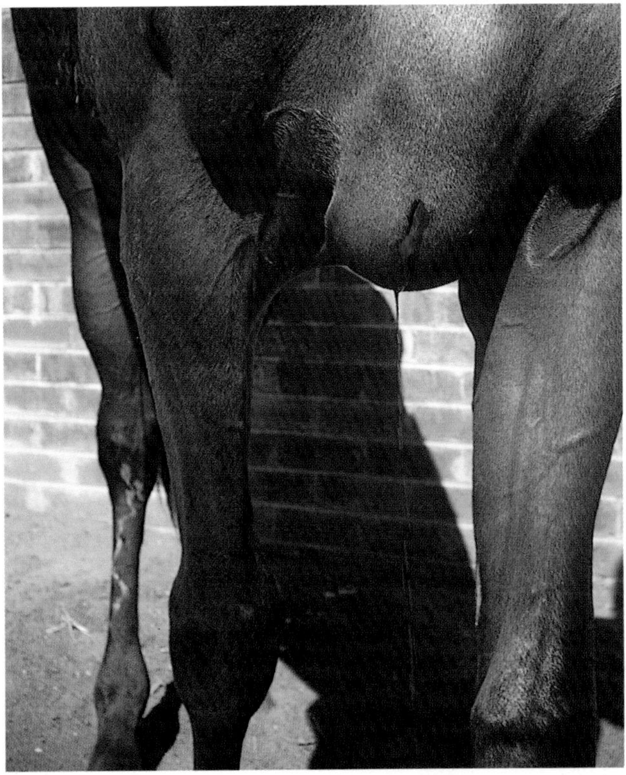

Draining a haematoma

CAUSES
Horse running into fence – crashing into doorway – falling over – being kicked by another horse – any blow that damages skin and underlying tissues severely enough to rupture local blood vessels – blood leaks into the surrounding tissues, forming a haematoma.

TREATMENT
In early formation of haematoma ice packs and cold hosing help stop bleeding and reduce swelling. If blood-filled cavity has formed – continue applying cold foments – call your veterinarian – he usually leaves haematoma for 4–5 days before draining it – allows ruptured vessel to seal itself off and bleeding to stop before cavity opened.

If haematoma of any size is not opened and drained, over several months blood may be converted into hard fibrous swelling that remains as permanent blemish.

# HEART DISEASE

The heart is a four-chambered, muscular pump, made up of special muscle fibres. The pumping action is controlled by electrical impulses released from a small node situated in the heart muscle, but this automatic control is over-ridden by other factors when the horse is excited or disturbed.

The function of the heart is to circulate blood to the numerous tissues and organs throughout the body. Basically, blood goes from the heart to the lungs where the red blood cells are replenished with oxygen and their waste products removed. The oxygenated blood then goes to the tissues and organs, where it exchanges oxygen for carbon dioxide and other waste products. It is then said to be deoxygenated blood; it travels back to the heart and is again pumped to the lungs, where waste products are removed and the blood reoxygenated.

SIGNS
Symptoms of heart trouble include poor performance during training, fatigue and poor exercise tolerance – horse has laboured, rapid breathing and rapid heart rate following moderate exercise – respiration and heart rate take a long time to return to normal after exercise. These signs not specific for heart disease but be suspicious if your horse exhibits them.

Heart murmur, detected with stethoscope – associated with incomplete closure of heart valves – when heart muscle contracts on a supposedly closed chamber, some blood leaks through the partially closed valves – adversely affects cardiac output, oxygenation of tissues, exercise tolerance and performance of horse.

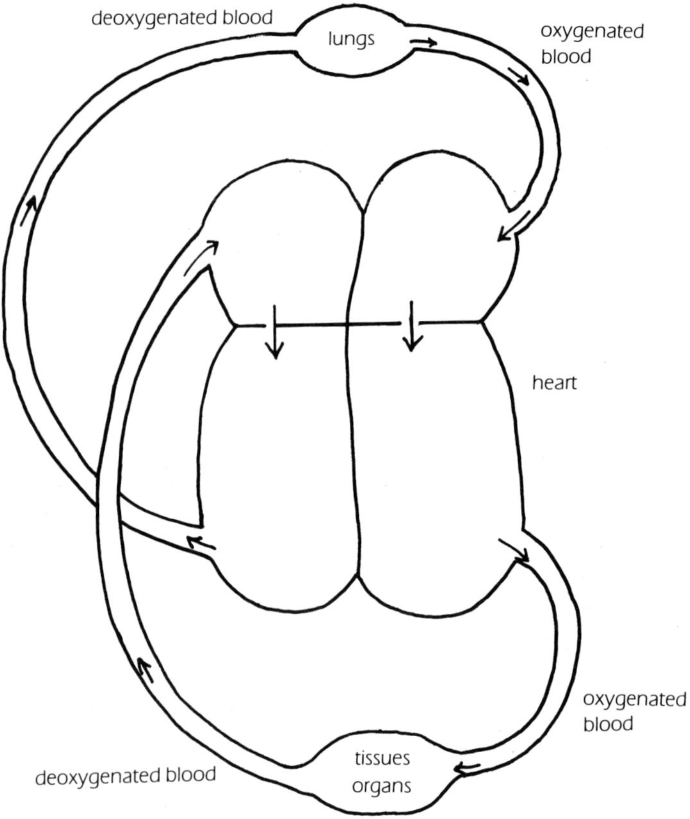

deoxygenated blood
lungs
oxygenated blood
heart
oxygenated blood
tissues organs
deoxygenated blood

Blood flow to and from the heart

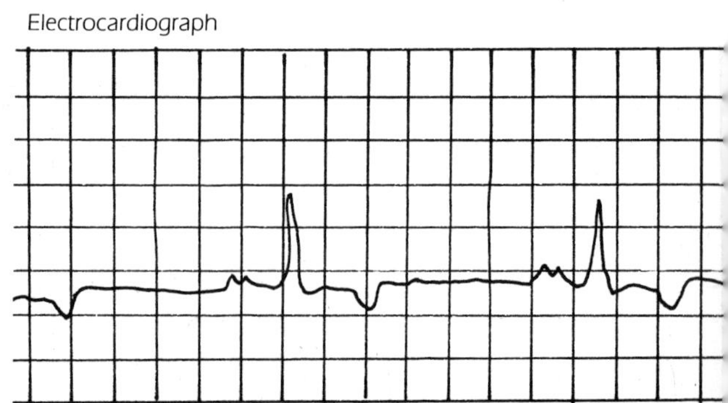
Electrocardiograph

Myocarditis or inflammation of heart muscle detected by your veterinary surgeon using an electrocardiogram – enables him to evaluate abnormalities in heart and to assess heart size. It is not an uncommon condition – seen in performance horses such as the polo, endurance, event and racehorse – some horses show signs of a good first-up performance when resuming after a rest or spell – the performances become progressively worse as horse competes more and more – in other cases, horse racing over a distance of 1200 metres may be in winning position at 1000-metre mark and racing keenly – in the last 200 metres it fades from a winning position to finish at tail of field.

CAUSES

Horse may be born with a heart defect – viruses and bacteria may also damage heart muscle and valves – unfit horse put into hard training too quickly or fit horse subjected to prolonged periods of stress may also suffer heart problem.

TREATMENT

If horse born with heart murmur or acquires murmur from damage to heart valve, no treatment is available – most of these horses lead a normal life, but some do not – author knows of a number of racehorses with heart murmurs that race and win.

If horse has myocarditis, consult your veterinary surgeon who will prescribe appropriate treatment. In training racehorse subject to myocarditis – get horse fit and at its peak a few weeks before the event – taper workload and keep horse as fresh as possible with light exercise prior to race – space races so that horse has plenty of time to recover as well as using them to help maintain horse's fitness – if horse requires a gallop before race, make sure it is at least 4 days away from the event, allowing horse and its heart muscle sufficient time to recover.

Horses with myocarditis often race better if nursed along during the race until 100 metres or so from finishing post and are then called on to make final sprint to line. They sometimes respond well to treatment and altered training methods – other horses with myocarditis become progressively worse with more exercise and racing.

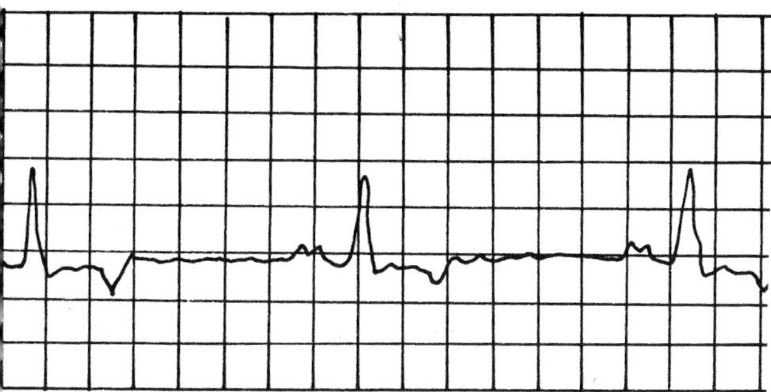

# HEATSTROKE

SIGNS
Sudden onset following hard work in hot, humid weather conditions, confinement in stables with poor ventilation, crowding in yards or floats with other horses – mucous membranes brick red – rapid respiration – dilated nostrils – heart rate rapid – patchy sweating – high temperature – staggers – collapse – unable to get up – convulsions – in some cases death.

CAUSES
Hard work in hot, humid weather – confined in a hot, humid environment with poor ventilation – often associated with restricted access to water.

TREATMENT
Cool horse down immediately – remove saddle or rug – cold hose – provide good ventilation and shade – hold ice packs on head – continue cold hosing until temperature returns to normal – provide cool water to drink on basis of little and often. Call your veterinarian who may give fluids and electrolytes intravenously and other drugs to counteract shock.

# HEAVES (Broken Wind)

This term is often erroneously used for horses that are roarers (see roaring, page 272). Correctly, the term refers to horses that have difficulty with expiration, i.e. breathing out, especially during and after exercise. Affected horses are of little use for work.

SIGNS
Appears in horses 5 years or older – signs appear gradually – most prominent sign is exaggerated and lengthy expiration especially during or after exercise – over a period of time breathing becomes difficult, even at rest – horse develops barrel chest to help compensate – wheezing associated with short, shallow cough is evident.

CAUSE
This disease is a chronic form of Bronchial Asthma or COPD (see page 170 for causes).

TREATMENT
Rest in a well-ventilated, dust-free stable is effective, coupled with putting horse out to pasture in good weather – dampening feed to keep level of dust at a minimum also necessary – in cases where air sacs in lungs have ruptured, nothing can be done.

Contact your veterinarian who can confirm diagnosis by listening to horse's chest with a stethoscope and by evaluating oxygen level of arterial blood.

# HEPATITIS

Hepatitis is inflammation of the liver and jaundice is associated with conditions of the liver or bile ducts. The horse has no gall bladder.

SIGNS
Jaundice (yellow discolouration of mucous membranes of conjunctiva, gums, etc.) – may be accompanied by high temperature – not eating – depression. Skin of white horses may show signs of yellowing.

CAUSES
Infection – obstruction of bile ducts – plant poisoning (plants containing pyrrolizidine alkaloids).

TREATMENT
Call your veterinarian who will take blood sample to evaluate cause of hepatitis – urine sample can also be useful in diagnosis – veterinarian will treat horse according to specific cause and symptoms.

# HOOF CRACK

SIGNS
Crack in hoof wall – short and shallow to long and deep – crack can start at ground surface of hoof wall or at coronary band – if depth of crack involves sensitive tissues, horse will probably be lame.

CAUSES
Trauma – drying out of hoof wall – excessive rasping of hoof wall – poor hoof care (trimming and shoeing).

TREATMENT
Can vary according to position, length and depth of crack – if crack starts at ground surface, treatment designed to prevent its expansion by putting shoe clips on either side, as well as rasping weight-bearing edge of hoof wall so that no pressure is borne by wall in the area of crack.

With both kinds of crack (i.e. starting at ground surface or coronary band) a groove should be burnt or filed at right angles to end of crack to stop its progress – if crack involves sensitive tissues it needs to be treated by a veterinarian, who will administer a tetanus and antibiotic injection and apply tincture of iodine locally to the crack.

Prevention includes trimming and reshoeing every 6 weeks – minimal rasping of hoof wall – daily hoof dressing (⅔ neatsfoot oil, ⅓ stockholm tar) – the use of boots to prevent damage to coronary band.

# HORMONAL IMBALANCE (mare)

The normal reproductive cycle of the mare is best determined by a pony teaser or stallion. The veterinarian can confirm the stage of oestrus.

SIGNS
During normal breeding season mare may not come into season regularly – fails to show signs of heat – is on heat or in season continuously – has irregular lengths of heat cycles. If any of these factors are obvious call your veterinarian to examine mare – he will establish whether or not she has hormonal abnormality.

CAUSE
Imbalance in hormone levels.

TREATMENT
Hormone therapy – this varies according to the type of hormonal abnormality.

# HORMONAL PROBLEMS (stallion)

SIGNS
Lack of libido – poor quality spermatozoa.

CAUSE
Hormonal imbalance.

TREATMENT
Contact your veterinarian – rest stallion showing lack of libido due to overuse – hormone treatment can be given with varying degrees of success – prolonged use of hormones (testosterone) may eventually cause reduction in size of testicles, resulting in permanently low libido.

I

# INFECTED PENIS AND PREPUCE

The male horse's genitalia are designed anatomically so that the penis is completely enclosed by the prepuce (sheath), except when the horse urinates or becomes sexually aroused. In its moist, warm, dark, waxy environment, with poor circulation and numerous folds and crevices, the penis is ideally suited for the growth and proliferation of bacteria.

## SIGNS

Creamy discharge from prepuce – irritation is indicated by rubbing or dropping out of penis – when penis extended surface is covered with heavy, waxy scales – the folds are inflamed and swollen and have an accumulation of pus – unpleasant odour associated with discharge.

## CAUSES

Poor hygiene is a primary cause of penis infections – if penis not cleaned regularly, scale, waxy secretions and debris accumulate in its folds and crevices and also in those of prepuce – foreign bodies such as grass seeds may also enter prepuce while horse is walking through long grass or herbage.

## TREATMENT

Place bucket of warm water, anti-bacterial soap such as chlorhexidene and clean towel nearby for use during treatment. Gently put hand into prepuce, take hold of head of penis and slowly pull it out – when it is fully extended, keep hold of it with left hand and wash it thoroughly, removing any debris – rinse well with clean water and dry with clean towel – if this is not done, any soap left on penis will act as an irritant, causing sensitive skin to become inflamed and susceptible to infection – if area is heavily infected, contact your veterinarian, who will give an antibiotic injection – smear a mild antiseptic cream inside prepuce and around penis – about once a month, the penis should be cleaned and coated with this cream, which acts as a lubricant and reduces bacterial contamination.

# INFECTED UTERUS (Metritis)

Infection is the most common cause of infertility in mares. Bacteria are harboured in the reproductive tract and pathogenic ones are known to cause infection of the uterus.

SIGNS
May or may not show vaginal discharge – failure to conceive or maintain pregnancy – normal reproductive cycle – more common in old mares with poor breeding history.

CAUSES
Windsucking through vagina can be common cause – more often seen in mares that have had numerous foals, with consequent loss of tone in lips of vulva – or in mares with sunken anus and vulva that slopes downwards and outwards. Most common bacteria in mare with infected uterus are *Streptococcus zooepidemicus*, *E. coli*, Pseudomonas and Staphylococcal species.

TREATMENT
Mares who windsuck or have structural defects of vulva should have lips of vagina stitched together – veterinarian performing

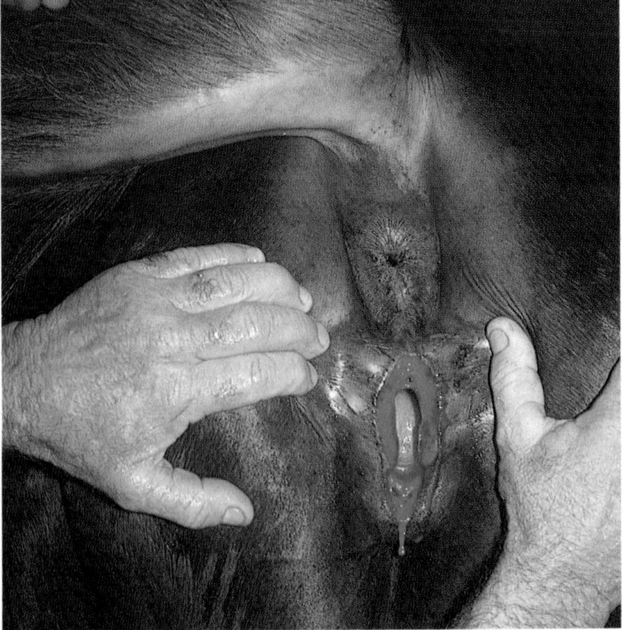

Caslick's operation: mucous membrane is trimmed from the lips of the vulva to prepare it for stitching

operation (Caslick's operation) allows room at end of vulva for mare to urinate – this operation prevents air contaminated with faeces and bacteria being sucked into uterus.

Racing fillies with poor conformation of vulva benefit from this surgical procedure.

Veterinary surgeon makes positive identification of infected mares by swabbing or clinically examining reproductive tract. Swabs can be taken routinely from mares in season or when infection suspected – if positive, veterinary surgeon's treatment will be to administer appropriate antibiotic – by injection or uterine irrigation at correct stage of oestrous cycle.

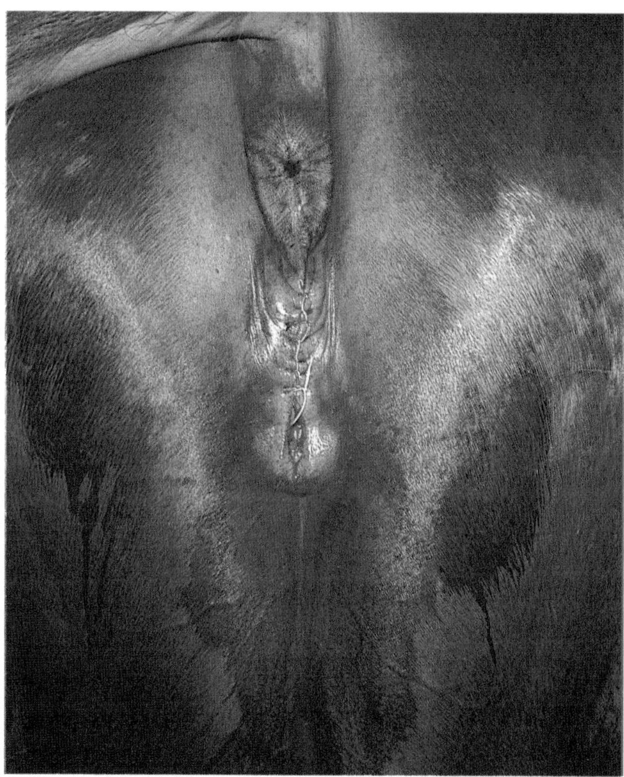

The lips of the vulva stitched together

# INFECTION: Unknown Origin

SIGNS
Lethargic, dull, not eating or eating only a little, temperature. No other signs.

CAUSE
Unknown infection.

TREATMENT
Call your veterinarian who will administer antibiotics providing he can find no other signs in a preliminary detailed examination – if horse responds to antibiotics then origin of infection is unimportant – if horse does not respond to the treatment within 24 hours then a further investigation by blood tests, urinalysis, etc, is necessary to localise type of infection and its site.

# ISOIMMUNE HAEMOLYTIC JAUNDICE

The most common jaundice found in newborn foals, this condition can be compared to Rh disease in human babies.

SIGNS
Occurs in new-born foal – sluggish – dull – weak – no longer suckles – lies down – rapid, shallow breathing (panting), especially after exercise – anaemic (pale gums and conjunctiva) – then gums and conjunctiva change to varying shades of yellow – after 24 hours urine dark brown – may collapse and enter coma.

CAUSE
Due to clash between antibodies in mare's colostrum and red blood cells in foal – end result destruction of foal's red blood cells – death follows if disease not arrested – remember foal is not born with this disease.

TREATMENT
Call veterinarian immediately – if foal less than 48 hours old prevent foal suckling mare – muzzle the foal or remove it – feed foal colostrum per foster mother, baby's bottle, stomach tube – mare should be milked out hourly – discard the milk – after 48 hours allow foal to return to mother to suckle naturally. Veterinary surgeon treats mild cases with antibiotics – more severe cases given blood transfusion.

Can be prevented – veterinarian gives pregnant mare blood test before foal born – if positive, no milk from that mare given to foal for first 48 hours – give foal colostrum from foster mother or from supply held in deep freeze for such emergency. Advisable to send mare to different compatible stallion for next service.

# J

## JOINT ILL

SIGNS

Heat, pain and swelling in affected joint(s) of new-born foal – lameness – stiffness in movement – temperature rise.

CAUSE

Arthritic condition caused by generalised infection (septicaemia) localising itself in one or more joints of new-born foal.

TREATMENT

Call veterinary surgeon – while awaiting his arrival, confine foal and mare to a clean box or yard where warmth and rest are available – check mare's milk supply to see that foal adequately fed – make sure mare is thoroughly clean around the vulva, udder and legs – wash with Hibiclens or similar preparation – apply supportive bandages to the affected joint(s) of foal – hot foment or poultice affected joint(s) with antiphlogistine.

To control joint ill: wash mare thoroughly after foaling – make sure foal given adequate colostrum – apply tincture of iodine on stub of umbilical cord of new-born foal – alternate foaling paddocks every two years and control parasites.

# K

## KIMBERLEY (Walkabout) DISEASE

SIGNS

Yawning – sleepiness – depraved appetite – irritability – unco-ordinated – twitching of head and neck muscles – walking in a straight line – may stand for hours pushing against immovable objects – reluctant to lie down – urine red to brown colour – mucous membranes may be jaundiced – over period of weeks extreme weight loss – eventually unable to get up – coma – death. Occurs in Western Australia and Northern Territory.

CAUSE

Poisonous native plant, *Crotalaria retusa,* found in low-lying areas of rivers subject to flooding in Kimberley district of Western Australia and Northern Territory.

TREATMENT

There is no treatment. Prevent by restricting access to the plant.

## KNOCK KNEES

SIGNS

Young foal with knee(s) bowing inwards.

CAUSES

Particular cause of limb deformities difficult to isolate – may be a single one or combination of several – generally, causes may be classified as nutritional, malpositioning of foal in mare's uterus, inherited genetic abnormalities or injury.

TREATMENT

Essential to treat deformity as soon as possible to remedy it – failing that, to stabilise it. It is always wise to check nutritional status of mare and foal – if necessary supplement their diet with vitamin and mineral supplement rich in calcium.

Confine foal to stable – hoof trimming is successful form of treatment in most cases – outside edge of hoof should be kept trimmed by rasping it repeatedly until leg is straightened – cases that fail to respond to this treatment should be referred to veterinarian – a metal staple may have to be inserted surgically on inside of knee to correct the problem.

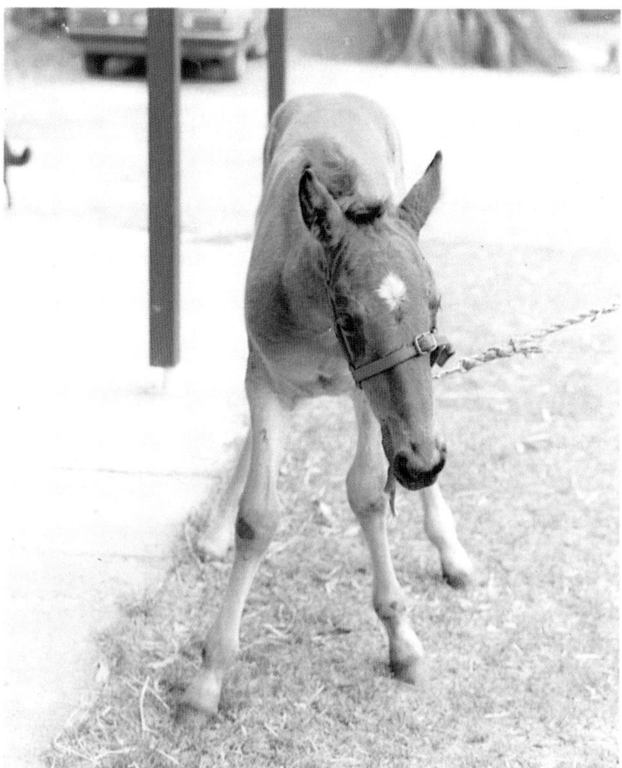

This foal has knock knees

# L

## LACERATED CHEEKS AND TONGUE

### SIGNS

Horse refuses food – slow in eating – excessive salivation – blood coming from mouth – quidding food, i.e. dropping food that has been partially chewed from mouth – lack of response to the bit such as pulling or hanging to one side – throwing head – swelling of cheeks which are painful to pressure.

### CAUSES

Mainly involves molars which are associated with grinding of food – action of chewing is an up-and-down movement as well as a side-to-side one – this action, coupled with fact that upper jaw is wider than lower jaw, results in outside edges of upper molars and inside edges of lower molars being ground to razor-sharp edge. Sharp edges of upper molars lacerate cheeks – lower molars lacerate tongue, causing glossitis, i.e. inflammation of tongue.

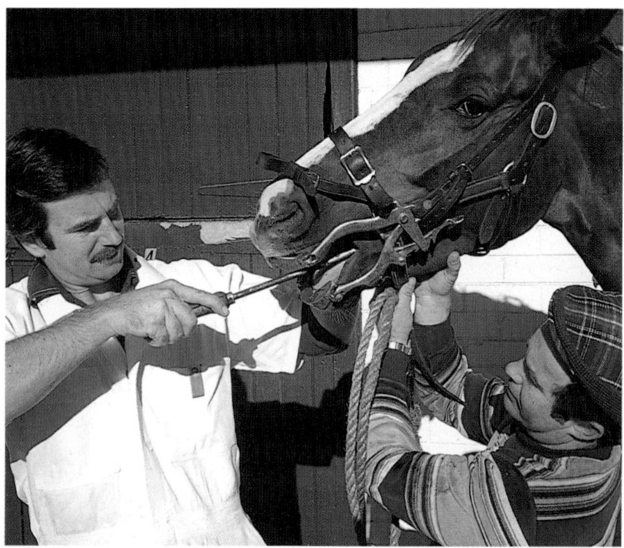

Rasping the molar teeth

TREATMENT

Call your veterinarian to do a detailed examination of mouth – can be done without a gag – a gag removes risk of being bitten – allows one plenty of time to feel and to look at teeth, to check tongue and inside of cheeks.

Sharp edges are removed by rasping or floating teeth with a long-handled rasp.

Teeth should be inspected every 4 months.

# LACERATIONS

SIGNS

Wound edges irregular – jagged and gaping – sometimes whole sections of skin and underlying tissue torn away – not usually acutely painful – haemorrhage variable, depending on type of blood vessels severed.

CAUSE

Probably most common type of wound – chief cause is barbed wire.

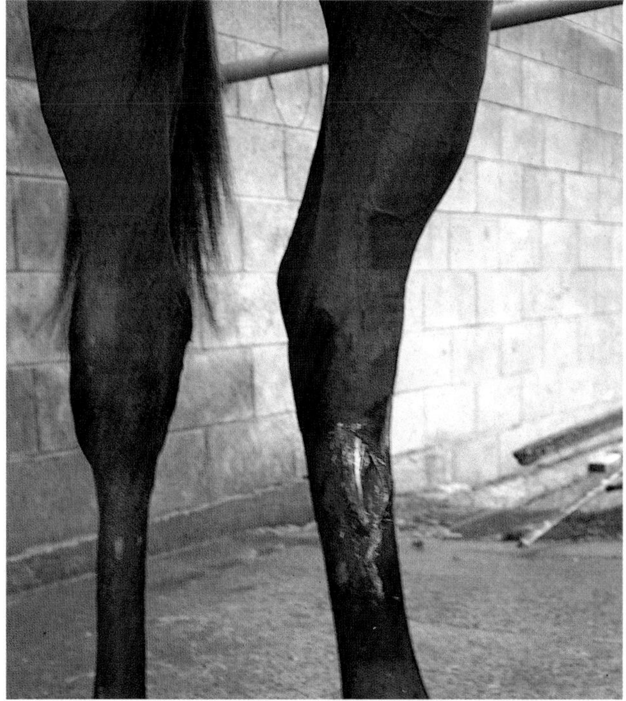

Laceration

### TREATMENT

Complicated – call your veterinarian for advice on stitching – if cannot be stitched, clean thoroughly – hose with fair water pressure or apply peroxide – remove any hair, dead tissue, foreign bodies – apply antibiotic powder, zinc cream or mild astringent to exposed flesh – avoid strong antiseptics as they can fail to destroy bacteria, irritate wound and destroy tissue cells necessary for healing.

If laceration on leg – cover wound with gauze – firmly apply Elastoplast bandage to hold gauze in position – firm bandage controls swelling – immobilises wound edges – stops production of proud flesh – leave on for 2 days if leg doesn't swell – a too tight bandage impairs blood supply – slows down healing – causes swelling of leg.

When bandage removed, it will be soggy and discoloured with discharge – odour probably offensive – this is normal if horse on good antibiotic cover. Hose wound clean – remove discharge, debris, etc. Continue similar treatment till fleshy tissue has filled in cavity to skin level. Only then, leave off bandage to allow air and sunshine to dry wound surface.

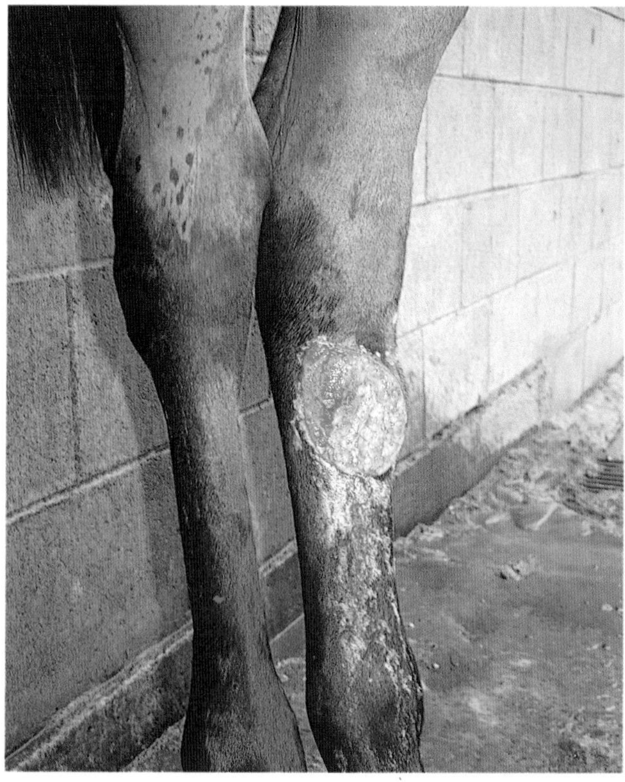

Proud flesh

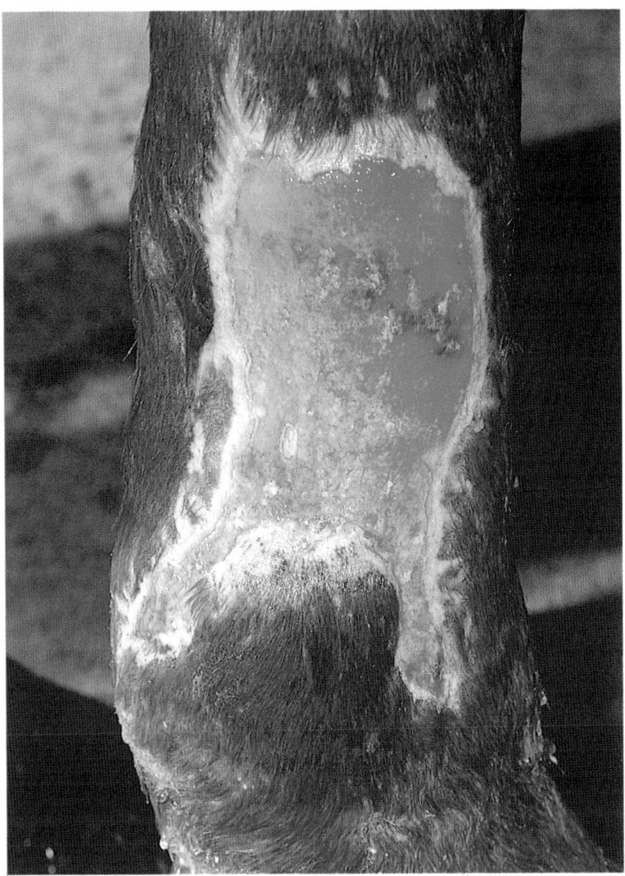

The light pink line around the wound indicates sensitive skin at the wound edge

If fleshy tissue raised above skin level – called proud flesh – must be cut back to allow skin to grow over wound – do this by applying copper sulphate solution to proud flesh – keep it away from sensitive skin at wound edge – do this day by day till flesh level with skin – skin should gradually close over wound. Excessive proud flesh should be cut back by veterinary surgeon. Confine horse to yard or stable – do not exercise until skin covers wound.

# LAMINITIS

See Founder (page 211).

# LAMPAS

Lampas is a swelling of the mucous membrane covering the hard palate behind the upper incisor teeth.

SIGNS
Swollen membrane of hard palate – if extends below level of tables of incisor teeth may cause discomfort when eating – horse may go off feed.

CAUSE
It may be associated with feeding or eruption of permanent incisor teeth.

TREATMENT
No special treatment required. The problem will rectify itself within few days. Any tooth irregularities should be corrected.

# LEG MANGE

Mites live on the surface of the skin. They inhabit primarily the fetlock region and the butt of the tail, but in severe cases can extend to other parts of the body. Long winter coats matted with dirt encourage the spread and development of mange.

SIGNS
Severe irritation confined mainly to legs below knees and hocks – may involve armpits, inner thighs, belly. Muzzle and nose may become involved by horse rubbing legs with its muzzle. Skin in affected areas is red – oozes serum which forms into hard crusts – in chronic cases skin forms thickened folds. Hair on legs becomes broken from constant rubbing – assumes moth-eaten appearance.

CAUSE
Chorioptic mites – up to 0.6 mm long – transmitted by direct contact between horses – rugs – grooming gear – harness – humans – dirty, damp, long winter coats encourage development and spread of mange mites – sick or debilitated horses and those suffering from vitamin/mineral deficiency are more susceptible.

TREATMENT
Definite diagnosis made by veterinarian following deep skin scrape and microscopic examination.

Isolate infected horses immediately – dip, spray or rinse horse in chlorinated hydrocarbons or organophosphorus compounds, e.g. Bayer Asuntol – use with caution – strictly follow directions for use – repeat treatment in 7 days.

Collect and burn loose hair and straw – treat affected stables with organophosphorus compounds – leave stable vacant for 4 weeks – don't use grooming gear or harness for 3–4 weeks.

# LICE

Lice infestation is most common in late winter and early spring. There are two kinds – biting and sucking lice. The biting louse is found on the body coat, the sucking louse in the long hair of the mane and tail. Lice are light grey in colour and 1–1.5 mm long. Lice that infect horses cannot survive on man or other animals, but biting lice can live for 10 days in loose hair shed by the horse.

## SIGNS

Severe irritation of skin – rubbing, biting and scratching – coat dull – some hair falls out – horse assumes motley appearance – long hair of mane and tail becomes matted – loss of condition – lice can be seen under good natural or artificial light if hair parted.

## CAUSES

Horses more susceptible to lice infestation if in poor condition – their coat is long – unkempt and dirty – they are kept in large numbers in a paddock, especially during infestation period.

## TREATMENT

Clip horse if body coat is long – any loose hair should be burned – spray horse thoroughly with Tiguvon, taking care to avoid nose, eyes and mouth – Tiguvon treatment should be repeated 3 weeks later.

To prevent lice: keep skin and coat clean by thorough and regular grooming – isolate any infected horses – treat grooming gear that has been used on infected horses with Tiguvon – brush loose hair from rugs used by infected horses – collect and burn hair – expose rug to sunlight – stables and yards should be cleaned of loose hair left by infected horses – all such loose hair should be burned.

# LOCKING OF STIFLE

In this condition the kneecap becomes fixed, locking the stifle in such a position that it prevents flexion of the hind limb.

## SIGNS

When stifle locked, leg assumes fully extended position with hoof bent backwards – when horse forced to move with stiff leg, front of hoof drags along ground – limb may remain locked in position of extension for hours or kneecap may be released every few steps, allowing leg to flex (bend) suddenly – often a snapping sound is heard as kneecap released – sudden release of kneecap with leg shooting forward can be mistaken for stringhalt (see page 284) by inexperienced observer.

## CAUSE

Problem is seen in all breeds and is inherited.

## TREATMENT

Contact your veterinarian – but in meantime if horse is backed or frightened, kneecap will often snap into position, releasing limb. Surgery offers a complete and permanent cure – done under local anaesthetic – results are immediate – horse walks away cured.

# M

## MASTITIS

SIGNS
Udder may be larger on one side than other – if infected, will be painful to touch, hot, swollen, hard, sometimes lumpy – milk may be thick and discoloured – difficult to express – if acute, mare will have high temperature.

CAUSE
Infection of udder.

TREATMENT
When treating mare for mastitis remove foal from her – apply hot and cold foments – milk mare manually – call your veterinarian – will treat her with antibiotics.

## MELANOMA

Melanomas are benign or malignant tumours of the skin.

SIGNS
Small (1 cm) to large (10 cm or more) dark lumps – may be located around anus or vulva, under tail, occasionally on or near eyelids – more frequently seen in old grey horses.

CAUSE
Unknown.

TREATMENT
Depending on tumour's size, nature and location and result of biopsy, veterinary surgeon will decide whether or not it should be excised surgically.

# N

## NAIL PRICK

### SIGNS

Most obvious is mild lameness shortly after shoeing – generally worsens each day – 3–7 days after being shod horse is acutely lame, just touching ground with toe of foot. Hoof wall is warm to touch – often pastern is swollen.

Severe pain exhibited by horse pulling foot away when it is squeezed with hoof testers or pincers or tapped with hammer – pain is worse when pressure is applied over offending nail. Removing shoe is often a painful procedure – carefully examine each nail and nail hole in hoof for moisture, blood or pus.

Arteries on either side of pastern supplying hoof pulsate more rapidly and strongly than normally.

### CAUSE

When shoeing, nail is placed incorrectly on inside of the white line or, when being driven, it crosses white line and penetrates sensitive tissues of foot – horse is referred to as having been 'pricked'.

### TREATMENT

Leave shoe off – clean around nail hole with tincture of iodine, removing debris and dirt – with clean hoof knife, enlarge hole to allow for proper drainage – soaking hoof in hot water for 10 minutes 3 times a day aids in healing and relieving pain – the water, with a teaspoon of an iodine-based solution added, should be just hot enough for the hand to tolerate it – level of water should not cover coronary band of hoof because it tends to swell and soften.

Fill hole with drawing agent such as magnesium sulphate paste, or paint hole with tincture of iodine – cover sole with Elastoplast to prevent further contamination from environment. The administration of antibiotics and tetanus antitoxin by your veterinarian are necessary precautions in treatment of puncture wounds.

# NAVICULAR DISEASE

The navicular bone is a boat-shaped bone lying close to the pedal bone within the hoof, under the centre of the frog. Horses with navicular disease put weight on the toe to protect the frog and heel from concussion. In some cases, over a long period of time, lack of frog pressure leads to contracted heels.

Navicular disease encompasses changes in the navicular bone, the navicular sac or bursa, and the flexor tendon that wraps around the navicular bone and attaches to the pedal bone. The disease is almost exclusively a front limb lameness.

## SIGNS

In early stages slight lameness that seems to fluctuate from one front foot to the other – as disease progresses horse steps short in both front legs, assuming a proppy, stilted gait, particularly at the trot – horse will often resent trotting and try to break into canter – when turning, rather than crossing its front legs, it will tend to shuffle round in order to lessen pressure on navicular bone.

## CAUSES

Inherited conformation such as short upright pasterns increase concussion and stress on navicular bone, bursa and deep flexor tendon – concussion associated with hard work on hard surfaces may cause navicular disease – improper trimming and shoeing may increase stresses placed on navicular bone.

## TREATMENT

Because of difficulty of accurate diagnosis and complexity of treatment, consult your veterinary surgeon if you suspect your horse has this disease.

Depending on severity of disease, treatment can involve corrective shoeing (raised heel and rolled toe shoes), which can give good results in horses used for pleasure riding but poor results in performance horses – anti-inflammatory and anticoagulant agents – desensitisation of affected part of foot by cutting certain nerves supplying area concerned. Whatever the treatment, range of success varies.

# NUTRITIONAL PROBLEMS (stallion)

There is very little information available on the relationship between nutrition and fertility in the stallion.

## SIGNS

Fat lazy stallion – laminitis (founder) – lack of libido – testicular degeneration and atrophy – poor quality sperm – decreased numbers of spermatozoa. If poor diet prolonged, these changes can be irreversible.

## CAUSES

Overfed stallions – vitamin A and vitamin E deficiency – severe undernutrition.

## TREATMENT

Vitamin A is essential for sperm production – green pasture is a source of carotene which is converted to vitamin A – drying process in exposing lucerne hay, clover and green herbage to sunlight and air helps destroy carotene – good hay is a source of vitamin A for 6–12 months after harvest.

Vitamin A can be stored in liver for 6–12 months – a stallion's daily requirement is 2000–5000 i.u. vitamin A per 50 kg body weight – ten times that amount can be toxic.

It has been claimed that vitamin E is important for increased libido and semen quality – requirement being 20 i.u. per 50 kg body weight – no scientific evidence to support claim.

The golden rule is always to give your stallion high quality feed but to regulate quantity to workload being undertaken. During stud season, depending on size of stallion and number of mares served, up to 12 kg of grain per day can be fed.

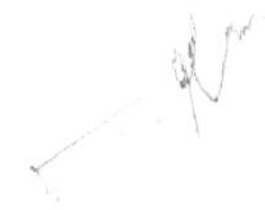

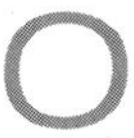

# ONCHOCERCIASIS

SIGNS
Circular areas of hair loss – about 2 cm in diameter – around head, neck and lower abdomen – scaly appearance of skin – itchiness – looks similar to ringworm.

CAUSE
Parasite *Onchocerca cervicales* – found in the skin – can be related to the eye condition, recurrent uveitis.

TREATMENT
Call veterinarian for a definite diagnosis – he will take skin biopsy for pathological examination and administer injections of anti-inflammatory drug to alleviate severe skin irritation and diethyl carbamazine to kill parasite.

# ORCHITIS

SIGNS
*Acute:* swelling of scrotum – stiff gait – one or both testicles may be involved – hot and painful if palpated – may refuse to serve mare (breed) – horse may have temperature rise.
*Chronic:* testes may be of normal size – insensitive to touch – feel harder than normal.

CAUSE
Usually due to infection – rarely due to trauma.

TREATMENT
If both testicles involved stallion more than likely will be infertile – contact your veterinarian – he will administer heavy doses of antibiotics for at least 5 days – if disease is in one testicle, castration of that one may be indicated to prevent spread of infection to the other.

# ORPHAN FOAL

When a foal loses its mother at birth or shortly after, it arouses our sympathy in a way that other animals seldom do. Because of strong emotional ties that develop between an orphan foal and its handler, the foal is often mismanaged to the point of being spoilt and subsequently grows into a mischievous, difficult weanling. A foal should be handled gently but firmly. If you want it to develop into a well-disciplined, obedient 2-year-old with a good temperament, its education must begin at birth.

## SIGNS

A foal loses its mother at birth or shortly after – also foal whose mother, for one reason or another, has no milk or cannot nurse her offspring.

## TREATMENT

Foal should be given at least 1200 ml colostrum, as soon as possible after birth – loses ability to absorb colostrum from its intestines after it is about 36 hours old.

*Bottle feeding:* foal should be fed every 3 hours for the first week of life – day and night – thereafter frequency of feeds should be decreased and amount increased – at 4 weeks old foal is fed 4 times a day. At each 3-hourly feed foal should receive 600 ml milk substitute – can be varied according to individual demand – substitute milk can be made up according to this formula: 300 ml cow's milk, 300 ml warm, boiled water, 5 ml (1 teaspoon) lime water and 1 teaspoon Glucodin. An alternative formula is 300 ml evaporated or powdered milk, 300 ml water and 1 teaspoon Glucodin.

Foals have ability to suck naturally – if foal rejects teat on bottle, place your index finger in its mouth – if it still does not suck, move index finger against roof of mouth and tongue – slowly replace index finger by teat on bottle once sucking has begun.

Disadvantage of bottle feeding is that it is time-consuming (cleaning bottle and teat and holding bottle while foal is feeding) and costly as far as labour is concerned.

*Foster mother:* in many cases a foster mother is not readily available when urgently required – some mares are good foster mothers – others will not readily accept orphan foal and may even reject it – mares that become a little fractious and unwilling in this situation can be calmed by use of a twitch or tranquilliser – wise to introduce orphan foal to foster mother with some caution so that no harm is done.

*Bucket feeding:* apart from foster mare, this is best form of feeding – easier and less time-consuming than any other and very effective.

At outset a little more time and patience are needed to encourage foal to feed from bucket – isolate it for a number of hours in a warm, safe environment until it wants some attention as well as being hungry – pour milk into plastic bucket with wide opening so that the foal will not balk at putting its head into it (a foal suckles naturally from its mother with its head up) – biggest problem in getting it to drink from a bucket is persuading it to suck with its head down – firstly, make it suck on your index finger with its head up, much as it does when suckling from the mare's teats – gradually direct its head downwards, foal still sucking on index finger, until its mouth is down in milk in bucket – withdraw the finger – with luck foal will continue sucking – if it doesn't suck after first attempt, go through same procedure again. Patience!

Milk prepared from a formula should be placed in bucket – keep at room temperature (though cold milk is quite suitable) – make it freely available to foal, in which case it will not overdrink – change milk and clean bucket thoroughly twice a day – hang bucket in a secure position at a height convenient for the foal to drink at will.

*Dry feeding:* once foal is drinking readily from bucket and is several days old – set up another bucket similar in shape and position containing about two handfuls of a readily digestible, milk-based, pelleted food. Encourage foal to eat pellets – place a few in the mouth and direct head to the bucket – once foal accepts pellets by eating them readily, make them freely available at all times – when foal is eating about 1 kg milk-based pellets per day, a grain-based pellet should be gradually substituted.

At 4 weeks of age, foal can be weaned completely off prepared milk formulae and fed dry pellets and good quality grains as well as limited quantities of hay.

*Stomach tube:* if foal is very weak and unable to stand, a tube can be passed into the stomach – preferably by veterinary surgeon – secure permanently in position – owner or stud groom can connect a funnel to tube and pour necessary nutritional requirements down tube every 3 hours – procedure should be continued until foal is strong enough to stand and suckle.

*Medication:* even if orphan foals have received colostrum, they should be given a course of antibiotics by veterinary surgeon as soon after birth as possible – this helps prevent infection.

# OSSELETS

This condition is most common in young racehorses, thoroughbreds and standard breds.

## SIGNS

Swelling appears just above or below front of fetlock – usually hard – pain on bending fetlock and lameness are present – swelling may only be thickening of joint capsule and soft tissue – or perhaps due to new bone growth.

CAUSES

Subjecting immature horses to a hard training and/or racing program – conformation faults of short or long upright pasterns increasing effect of concussion on front of fetlock joint.

TREATMENT

Rest essential. Cold hosing – firm application of bandages soaked in Epsom salts and iced water will help reduce inflammation and swelling. Call veterinarian – he will prescribe appropriate treatment that may involve X-ray and radiation therapy.

Preventive measures can be taken by corrective trimming of feet of horses with long or short upright pasterns – allow toe to grow longer and lower heels by trimming and rasping. Allow young horses plenty of time to mature – check horse's diet for correct balance in calcium–phosphorus ratio.

# OTITIS EXTERNA

This is an inflammation of the external ear canal.

SIGNS

Horse rubbing ear – shaking head – affected ear droops (not erect) – sensitive to putting on bridle – head may tilt to affected side – ear very sensitive to touch – may be odour and fluid, purulent discharge.

CAUSES

Foreign body, e.g. grass seed – infection, e.g. fungal or bacterial – trauma, e.g. laceration.

TREATMENT

Apply twitch to nose – clean ear thoroughly with cotton buds and Otoderm – call your veterinarian – will look into ear with an oroscope and check cause. Ear drops containing antibiotic, anti-inflammatory, antifungal agents are usually prescribed and effective. Ear canal poorly designed for drainage, so thorough cleaning is just as important as ear drops – over-zealous cleaning can aggravate an already existing problem or create a problem – horses with healthy ear canals do not require routine cleaning.

# OVER-REACHING (Forging)

SIGNS
Hind foot steps on heel of forefoot on same side – often toe of hind foot steps on heel of shoe on forefoot, pulling it off.

CAUSES
Faulty conformation (long legs, short body) – poor co-ordination associated with fatigue – poor trimming and shoeing slowing breaking action of front feet.

TREATMENT
Front leg is made to move faster than hind leg by shortening toe of front foot and by rolling toe of shoe and raising heel – crease of shoe removed to reduce friction – action of hind feet can be slowed down by lengthening toe and lowering heel of hoof.

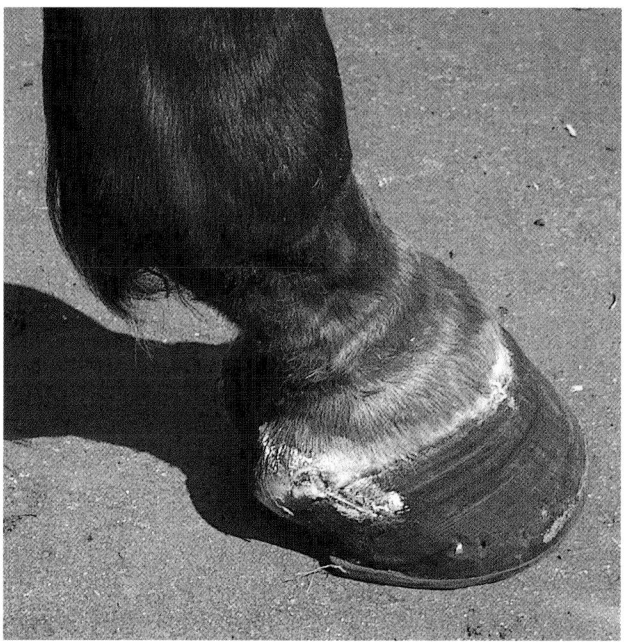

Over-reaching: a wound on the coronary band from the hind foot on the same side

# P

## PARASITES (Worms)

All horses have worms, although the young and old are most susceptible. Stables, yards, paddocks and wherever the horse passes manure are contaminated with worms and worm eggs. The worms and migrating larvae can cause damage ranging from temporary anaemia to death from a ruptured bowel.

SIGNS
Weight loss – dull harsh coat – poor appetite – pot belly – pale mucous membranes of eyelids and gums – tail rubbing – reduced performance – poor stamina – diarrhoea – colic – coughing in young foals – botfly eggs on coat.

Many healthy looking horses have worms – none appear in manure if worm burden not heavy. Signs alone do not indicate horse has worms – other health problems e.g. poor nutrition, irregular teeth give rise to similar signs.

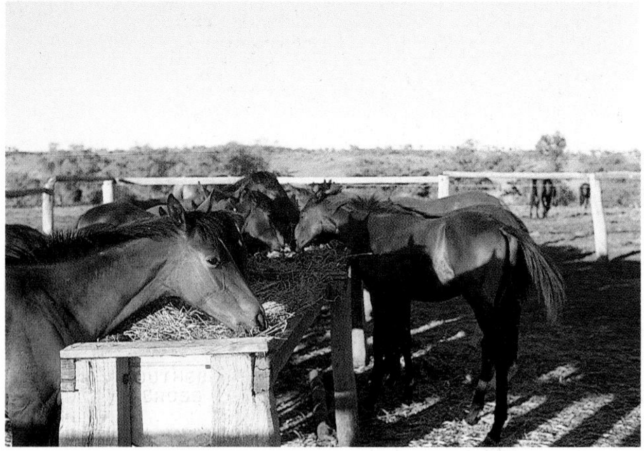

Worm prevention — feeding foals from a crib rather than off the ground

## CAUSES

Types of Worms

| Worm | Length | Colour | Shape |
|---|---|---|---|
| Habronema (large stomach worm) | 2 cm | White | Thin |
| Large strongyle (red worm) | up to 5 cm | Reddish | Thin with tapered ends |
| Small strongyle (red worm) | up to 2.5 cm | Reddish | Thin with tapered ends |
| Roundworm (milkworm) | up to 40 cm | White | Spaghetti-like |
| Bots | 1 cm | Brown to red | Grub-like |
| Pinworm | up to 10 cm | White | Whip-like |
| Tapeworm | 4 to 8 cm | Off-white | Flat |
| Strongyloides (threadworm) | 8 to 9 mm | | Thread-like |

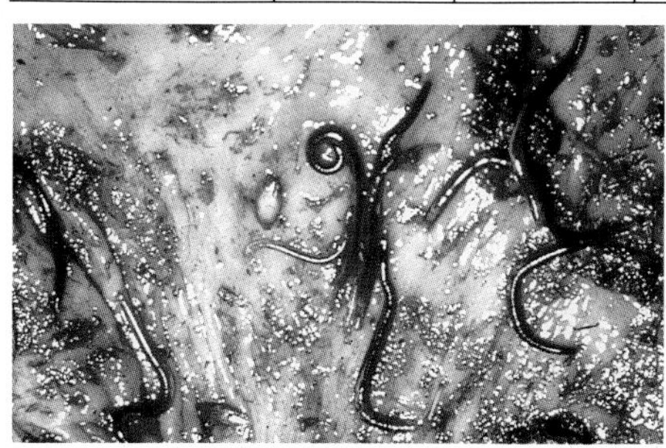

Large strongyle (red) worm

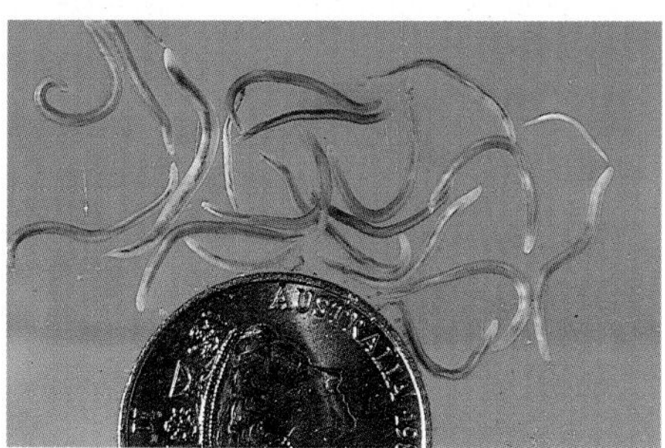


Small strongyle worms next to a one cent coin

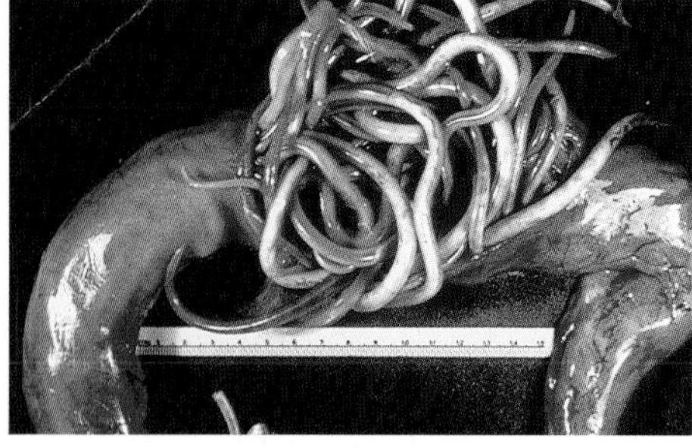

Roundworm (milkworm)

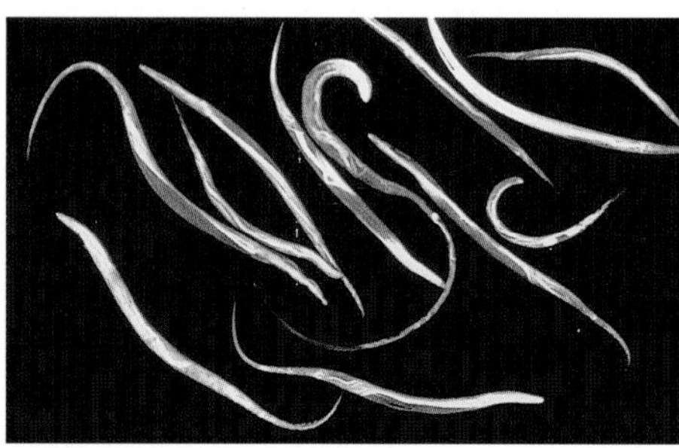

Pinworm

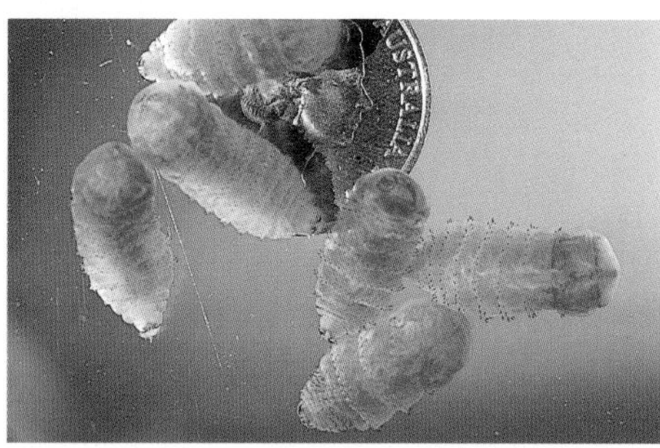

Botfly larvae

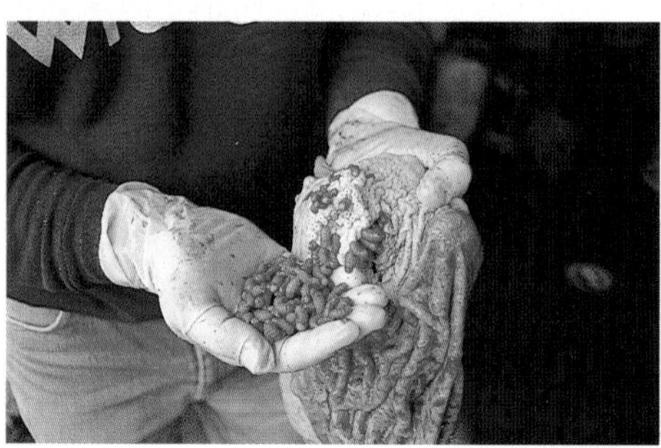

Bots in the stomach

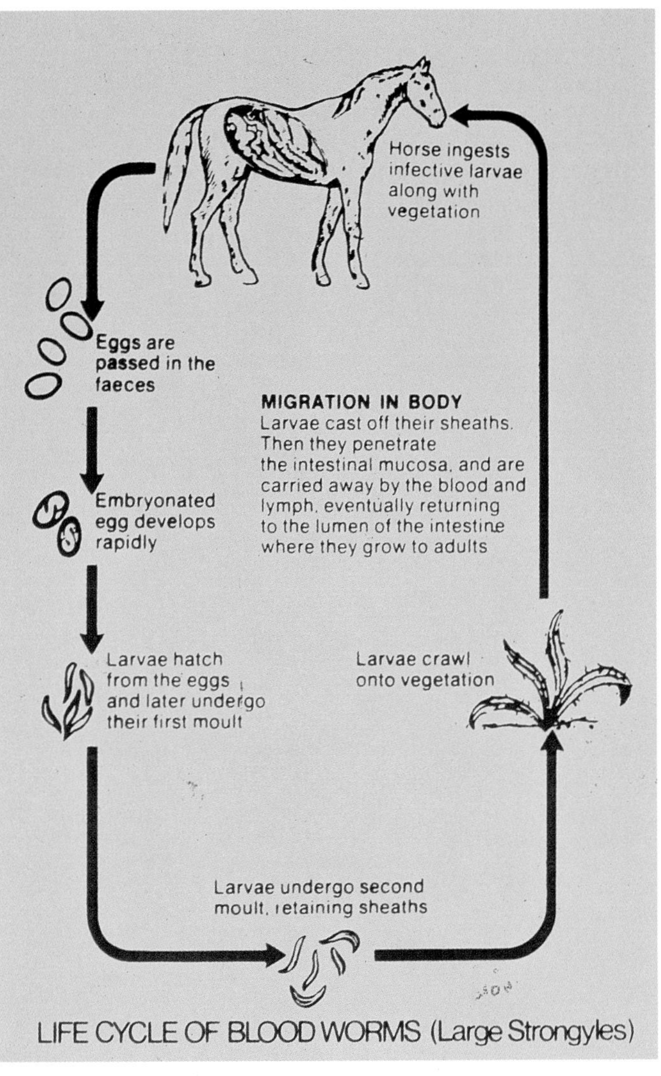


LIFE CYCLE OF BLOOD WORMS (Large Strongyles)

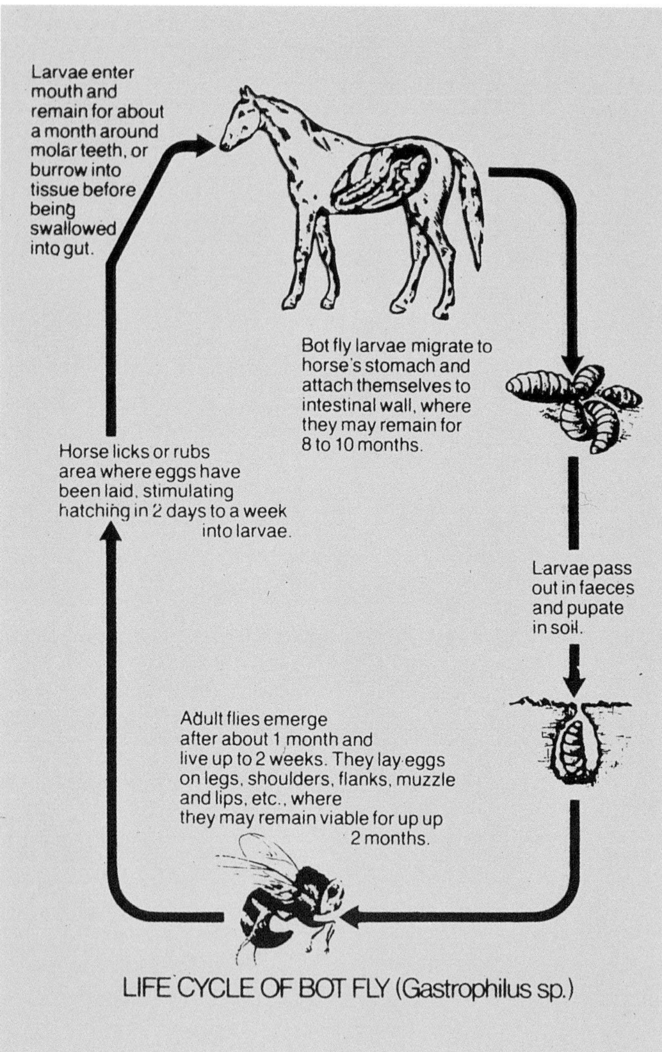

LIFE CYCLE OF BOT FLY (Gastrophilus sp.)

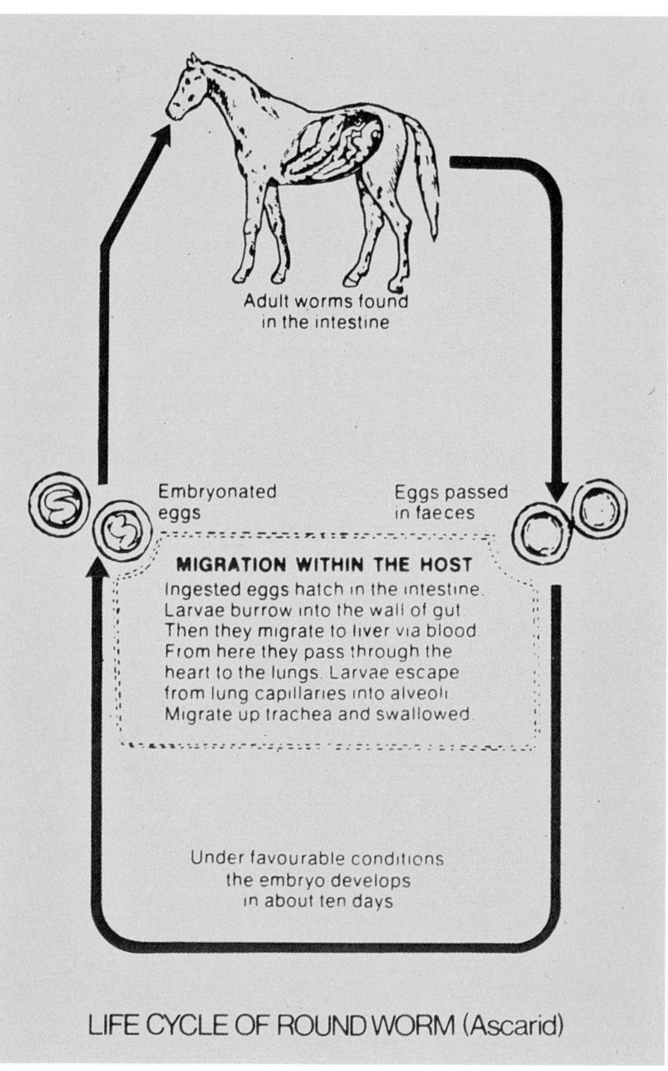


LIFE CYCLE OF ROUND WORM (Ascarid)

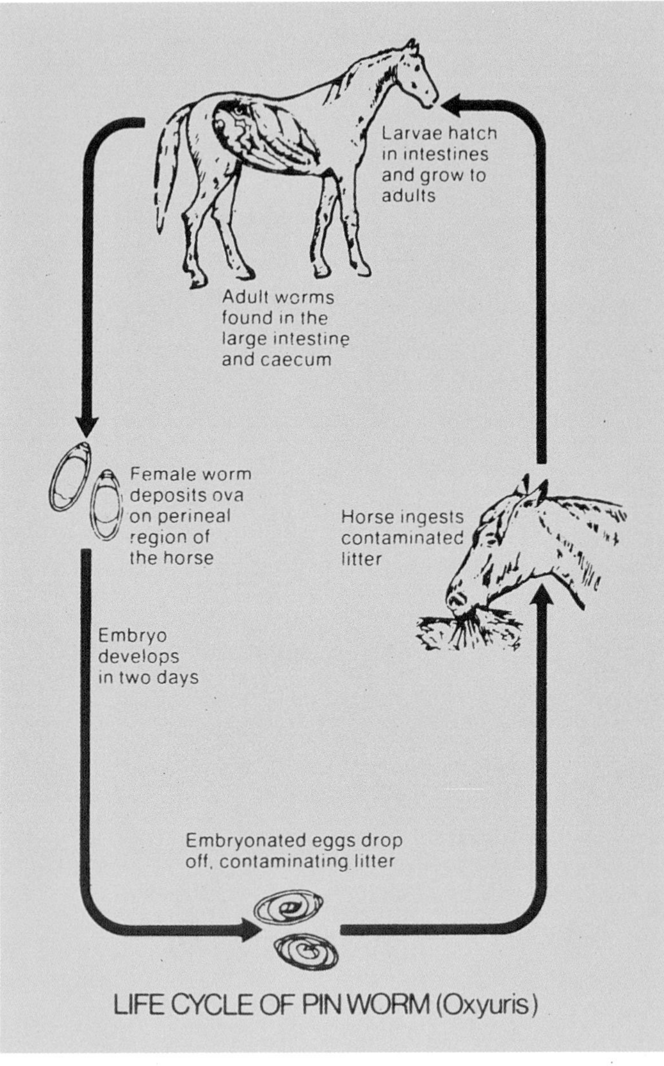


LIFE CYCLE OF PIN WORM (Oxyuris)

## TREATMENT

*Three approaches:*

- seek veterinarian's advice based on signs and symptoms of horse;
- have horse's manure (one ball) tested in veterinarian's laboratory to establish worms present, their type and burden;
- owner drenches the horse and checks improvement, if any – often long process and condition of horse may deteriorate while awaiting result.

*Methods of worming:*

- most efficient and direct method is stomach tube – should only be used by veterinarian or trained personnel. Pellets and granules in feed convenient and easy – make sure horse eats them. Worm pastes convenient and relatively easy to administer. Remember worming preparations only effective against adult worms in intestines and some worms have developed resistance to certain worming preparations – migrating immature larvae in other parts of body at time of worming not affected. As a precaution have manure sample tested by veterinarian 6 weeks after worming – note pinworm eggs usually not in manure.

*Worming program:*

- Worm pregnant mares every 6 weeks – final worming 4 weeks before foaling – do not use organo-phosphate compounds in last 3 months of pregnancy.
- Worm mare and foal every 6 weeks after foal 6 weeks old and until weaned. Foal can be infected with threadworm – via mare's milk – during first few weeks after foaling.
- Worm non-pregnant mares – weanlings – yearlings – teasers – stallions – every 12 weeks.
- Have laboratory tests done on manure samples twice a year.
- Worm all horses at same time – good idea – mares coming on to stud worm on arrival – keep in separate paddock for 3 days.
- Early spring – late autumn – best time to worm for bots.
- Ponies and horses in spelling paddock worm 4 times a year – manure test twice a year.
- Racehorses, hunters, event horses on return to stable from spelling should be wormed.
- If worms evident in droppings after treatment – repeat treatment in 4 weeks time.

*Management for prevention:*

Do not feed horses off ground – provide feed bins, water troughs, hay racks – worm eggs and larvae thrive on moist, muddy areas around dams – don't let water troughs overflow – fence off swamp areas or drain them – harrow paddocks where horses tend to gather around feed and water troughs.

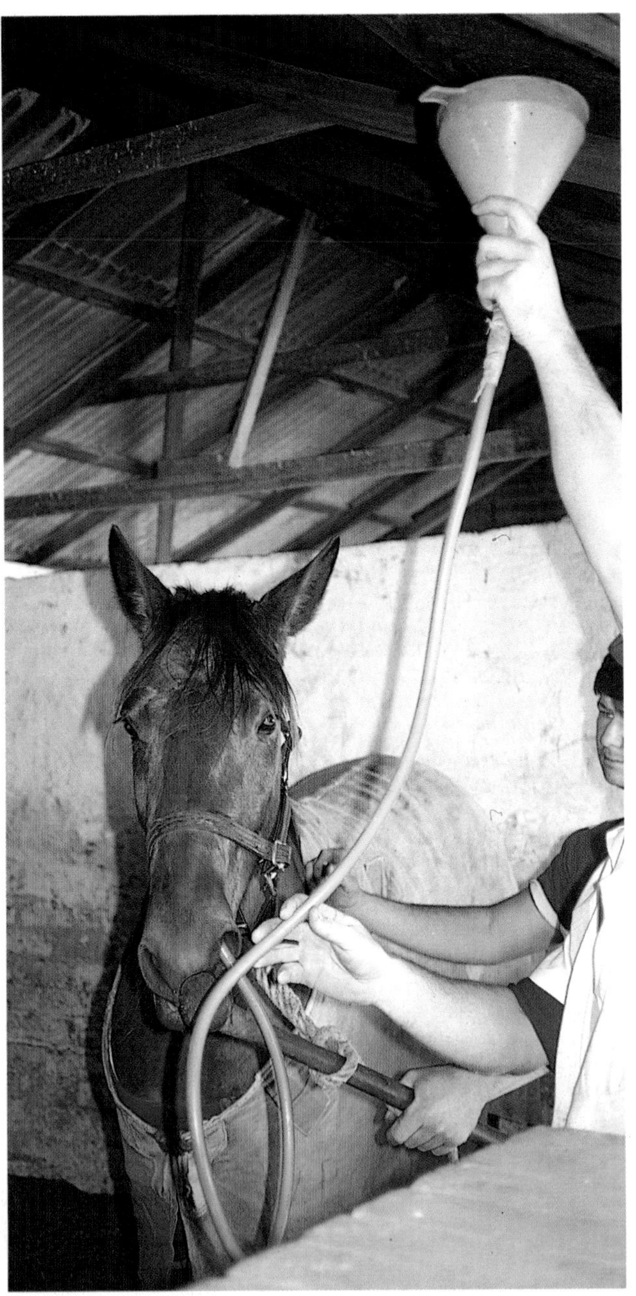

Worming via a stomach tube

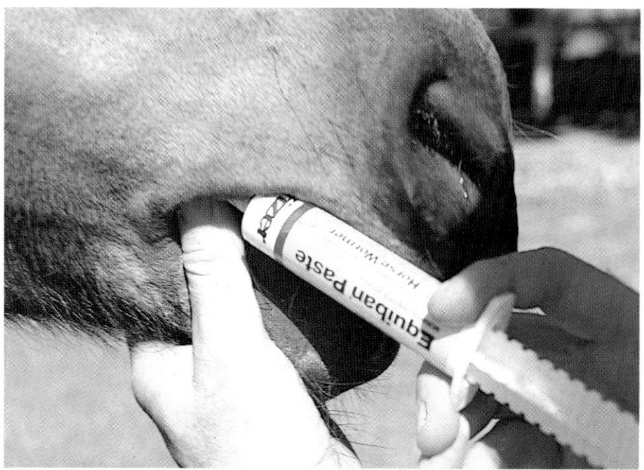


Administering worm paste

Pick up and dispose of manure in yards – slash long grass to expose manure to sun – kills worm eggs – spell paddocks and yards for 3 months from horses – rotate with cattle. Overcrowding results in heavy contamination – horses pick up more worm eggs – especially grazing closer to ground. Pick up manure and soiled bedding during day – put hay in nets, not on floor – clean feed bins and water buckets every day – automatic watering device helpful.

Concrete floors best – easy to clean – can be hosed and disinfected. Solid flyproof dung bin necessary – heat from combustion kills worm eggs – control fly activity with wire screens and baits. Wash and groom horse regularly – removes unseen eggs from coat – pinworm eggs found around base of tail – clipping and botfly knife also helpful in removing bot eggs.

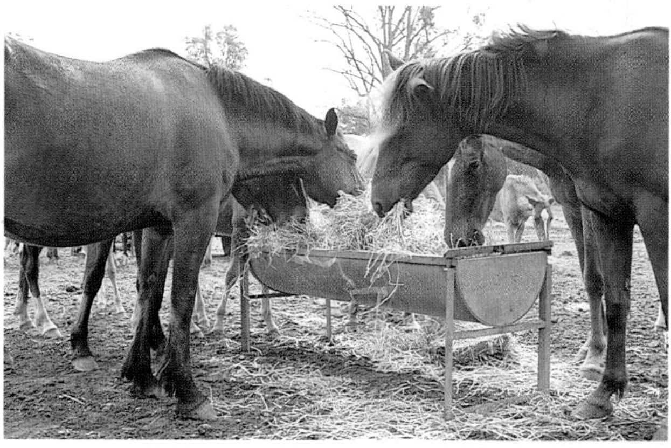

Feed horses from trough to prevent worms

# PATENT URACHUS

SIGNS
Urine leaks from stump of navel cord – flow increases when foal strains to urinate – often wet patch around umbilical stump.

CAUSE
When foal is in mare's uterus, urine produced by foal is discharged through a small fine tube in umbilical cord (urachus) into a membranous bag (allantoic sac) – when foal born and umbilicus breaks the urachus usually closes – not uncommon in newborn foals for urachus not to close completely.

TREATMENT
Call your veterinarian. Antibiotic cover for 5 days should be administered. Clean area thoroughly – cauterise navel stump daily with solution containing 10% iodine or silver nitrate until drip ceases. Dampness around umbilical stump makes it susceptible to infection leading to joint ill, septicaemia, etc.

# PAWING

SIGNS
Horse constantly paws ground – digs large holes – mostly near doorways – wears away toe of hoof.

CAUSE
Horse doesn't want to be confined – has excess energy.

TREATMENT
Put horse in larger yard or paddock – if unavailable put horse in stable with concrete floor – shoe horse to protect toe.

# PEDAL OR NAVICULAR BONE FRACTURE

Pedal bone fracture is more common in standard breds than thoroughbreds. A fracture of the navicular bone may be due to its weakening from chronic navicular disease.

SIGNS
Acute lameness immediately after race – affected hoof often held off ground – severe pain when hoof tapped with hammer or pressure applied to sole with hoof testers. If fracture of pedal bone

is through the wing, the horse in many cases will show signs of improvement after 48 hours stall rest. If fracture extends into coffin joint or if navicular bone is fractured, acute lameness and pain persist longer than 48 hours. Often no indication of swelling in leg above hoof.

### CAUSES

Normally occurs in performance horses – result of speed, concussion, hard and uneven track surfaces in conjunction with horse placing its foot awkwardly when fatigued – occasionally pedal bone fractured by foreign body penetrating through sole.

### TREATMENT

X-rays by your veterinarian essential to confirm and differentiate which bone is involved, position and extent of fracture.

If fracture involves pedal bone but does not extend into coffin joint, a bar shoe with quarter clips to limit hoof expansion, changed every 6 weeks over a period of 7 months, will often result in fracture healing.

If fracture of pedal bone extends into coffin joint, it usually heals in horses under 3 years of age using a bar shoe with quarter clips for 7 months followed by 6 months of complete rest. In horses over 3 years of age most successful treatment is surgery using a screw to compress fractured ends together.

Fracture of navicular bone will not heal completely, rendering horse useless for racing or performance-type events. A nerve supplying navicular bone and surrounding area may be severed to alleviate intractable pain and allow limited use of horse.

## PEDAL OSTEITIS

This condition is an inflammation of the pedal bone. Associated with it is demineralisation of the pedal bone and the formation of a roughness on its outer edge.

### SIGNS

Lameness sometimes present in front feet – other times absent – often difficult to tell if in right front leg or left front leg – as condition progresses, lameness obvious in all gaits – characterised by a short step.

### CAUSES

These include an inherited conformation that increases amount of concussion on pedal bone – concussion associated with hard work on hard surfaces – poor hoof care.

### TREATMENT

Consult your veterinarian. Treatment and its success vary according to severity and distribution of inflammation in pedal bone – treatment may involve rest, corrective shoeing, anti-inflammatory agents, a calcium supplement in diet or neurectomy (i.e. denerving).

## PERITONITIS

The membrane lining the abdominal cavity and covering the intestine is known as the peritoneum. Inflammation of the peritoneum is called peritonitis. Horses have a large area of peritoneum so peritonitis is a serious disease.

### SIGNS

Abdominal discomfort – pain – tense abdominal muscles – reluctance to lie down – severe depression – grunting associated with breathing or when forced to move – loss of appetite and weight – dehydration.

### CAUSES

Common cause is penetration of abdominal wall by sharp object such as broken fence rail. Another is rupture of stomach or intestines – contents spill into abdominal cavity – usually results in fatal peritonitis.

### TREATMENT

Call your veterinarian immediately – while waiting treat horse as if suffering from shock (see page 37). Preventive treatment includes elimination of sharp protruding objects from stable wall, fences, etc. – remove sharp objects such as rails, bailing wire from where horses graze – provide a systematic worming program – remember: bots can cause perforation of stomach wall.

## PLEURISY

The pleura is the membrane covering the lungs and lining the inside of the chest cavity. Pleurisy is inflammation of the pleura. When inflamed, in the early stages, the pleura may be dry, developing later into an exudative pleurisy when the pleura produces excessive fluid.

SIGNS
Sudden onset – temperature – not eating – lethargic – rapid shallow respiration – stands rather than lies down – doesn't want to move or turn round – short shallow cough. If you listen to chest with your ear you may hear a dry rasping sound. Tapping chest with your fingers may reveal a horizontal line of dullness – level of horizontal line varies depending on volume of fluid produced by pleura – if you listen to chest below horizontal line, respiratory sounds are dull or non-existent – swelling may appear under chest and in lower limbs. Death is not uncommon 2–3 weeks after onset of symptoms.

CAUSE
Often develops in association with pneumonia or a penetrating injury.

TREATMENT
Contact your veterinarian. X-ray will show if there is fluid in chest – withdrawal of fluid from chest and analysing it in laboratory will confirm diagnosis. Early treatment assures a better chance of survival – includes antibiotics, treatment for pain and drainage of fluid.

Future usefulness of horse doubtful following exudative pleurisy, due to formation of adhesions.

# PNEUMONIA

This is an infection or inflammation of lung tissue, often seen in foals and in debilitated, stressed or old horses.

SIGNS
Vary with suddenness of onset and volume of lung tissue involved. Generally, horse off its food – lethargic – respiration rapid and shallow – often a cough, nasal discharge and high temperature – breath may have foul odour – if you place your ear to chest, moisture may be detected as horse breathes in and out – the horse will stand in one place not wanting to move or lie down – in many cases, nostrils flared.

CAUSES
Viruses – bacteria – parasites – inhalation of foreign material. A stomach tube passed incorrectly by an untrained person into windpipe and fluid poured down the tube, passing directly into lungs, causes acute pneumonia – horse contracting pneumonia in this way usually dies or suffers permanent damage to lung tissue – rendering it useless for riding. Many predisposing causes of pneumonia – travelling – overcrowding – malnutrition – exhaustion – all lower horse's resistance to infection.

### TREATMENT

Keep in mind good nursing is essential part of any treatment. Consult your veterinary surgeon immediately – if treatment delayed or inadequate, 50% of affected horses probably die or suffer from permanent lung damage.

Place horse in well-ventilated, draught-free stable – keep its temperature as even as possible by rugging or by removing rug if temperature very high. Fresh water and nutritious, palatable feed should be available to encourage eating and drinking – electrolytes in feed or water are important to prevent dehydration. No exercise should be given for 4 weeks from time of apparent recovery, otherwise pneumonia could recur.

# POISONING

If a horse dies suddenly with no obvious signs of the cause, poisoning may be suspected. Poisoning can be identified conclusively only after a detailed post-mortem and laboratory tests of tissue samples from the body. If a sample of the stomach contents can be collected and sealed in a screw-top jar, it will be helpful in identifying the poison or plant ingested.

### SIGNS

General signs: depression – off food – dehydration – weight loss – laboured breathing. Specific signs: snake or insect bites usually cause swelling found on legs or head – salivation – diarrhoea – abdominal pain – twitching muscles – excitability – wobbling – paralysis – convulsions – coma.

### CAUSES

Snake bite, plants, chemicals, insects. Plant poisoning not common – horses tend to be selective in grazing – mineral poisoning rare because of regulation controls on use and disposal – e.g. arsenic – pesticide poisoning such as organocompounds uncommon in horse. Horses exposed to poisoning usually by accidental contamination – feed – pastures – water – or by accidental overdose when drenched for internal parasites.

### TREATMENT

Contact your veterinarian immediately. If poisoning due to something ingested give horse 5 litres mineral oil by mouth – don't give if signs of diarrhoea. If horse hyperexcitable, wobbly, paralysed – provide plenty of straw for bedding to prevent injury – place horse in dark, quiet stable – supply water containing electrolytes to prevent dehydration – if shock setting in, keep horse warm with rug. Check feed, pasture, water supply.

If snake bite – kill and keep snake for identification – apply broad cotton bandage tightly over and 7 cm either side of bite – ice pack or cold hose site of bite where bandage cannot be applied, e.g. muzzle – treat horse for shock (see page 37). Keep horse quiet as possible – movement will stimulate circulation of poison – ask the veterinarian to come to the horse.

# POLL EVIL

The poll is the prominence between the ears, indicating where the horse's spine joins the skull. Above and behind the prominence is a fluid-filled sac or bursa. If this becomes inflamed or infected and swollen, the condition is known as poll evil.

SIGNS
Tenderness around poll – may be noticed when putting on bridle – a painful, well-defined or diffuse, ill-defined swelling may be seen – stiffness in head movement – pus discharge in mane.

CAUSES
Infection can cause poll evil as can trauma, e.g. headband of bridle or headstall rubbing skin – horse rearing and hitting the back of head against hard object such as roof rafter. In few cases no observable evidence that infection or trauma is cause.

TREATMENT
Clip all hair well away from swollen area so that any discharge will not mat hair – otherwise, treat as for fistulous withers (see page 203).

# POST-FOALING METRITIS

The excretion of small amounts of clear, serous discharge, sometimes tinged with blood, is normal for the mare up to a week after foaling.

SIGNS
Temperature rise – lethargy – off food – 12–24 hours after foaling there is bloody brown or creamy yellow discharge from vulva – constant drip of blood – laminitis (see page 211) may be evident.

CAUSES
Tears, bruising and swelling of vulva – vagina and cervix susceptible to infection – retention of placenta or portion in uterus may lead to infection (metritis).

TREATMENT

Call veterinarian – he will administer antibiotics and anti-inflammatory agents, and take swab to identify type of infection and appropriate antibiotic.

# PREMATURE FOAL

Since the premature foal is not fully developed, it experiences greater difficulty in coping with the external environment than the normal foal. Some premature foals can stand and suckle (usually those who are 2–3 weeks premature) but some cannot (usually 5 weeks or more premature). Sparse body hair covering, such as in the mane and tail, is evident in many premature foals.

SIGNS

Premature foals are born before they are fully developed in mare's uterus – foals born after spending less than 330 days in uterus are classified as premature.

CAUSES

Hormonal – infection – unknown.

TREATMENT

Provide foal with warmth and protection from environment. Call your veterinarian whether or not foal can stand and suckle – will probably give foal an injection of antibiotics – if foal unable to stand and suckle an intravenous drip containing fluids and electrolytes will be given and stomach tube will be secured in position – actual feeding of colostrum through the tube can be done by the owner, stud groom or breeder – stomach tube can be left in position so that feeding can be continued until foal can stand and shows signs of suckling.

# PSYCHOLOGICAL PROBLEMS (mare)

SIGN

During normal breeding season mare shows no signs of heat (oestrus).

CAUSES

Mare may dislike colour of teaser – upset by strange environment – anxious about absence of new-born foal – worried about separation from another mare that she has strong attachment to.

TREATMENT

Identify the basic cause – take steps to counteract.

# PSYCHOLOGICAL PROBLEMS (stallion)

SIGNS AND CAUSES

Masturbation – reflected sometimes in lack of libido and poor quality semen – rejection of mare because of her colour, size, age, odour or some other factor obscure to handler – accepts and serves another mare vigorously – poor initial training and handling.

TREATMENT

To prevent masturbation a stallion ring is fitted onto flaccid penis – head of penis stops ring from slipping off – important that ring fits snugly but not too tightly – otherwise blood circulation to head of penis may be impaired with disastrous results.

To encourage the stallion to serve the mare, the stallion handler should be very patient and aware of stallion's idiosyncrasies and act accordingly.

# PUNCTURE WOUNDS

SIGNS

Hole in sole of foot or skin – variable size – neat or ragged edge – variable tissue damage under skin – generally painful – may or may not be bleeding.

CAUSES

Occur frequently, e.g. puncturing of sole by horseshoe nail left lying in yard – penetration of skin by wire or splinter when horse rubs against fence.

TREATMENT

Check wound to see no foreign body left in it – clean puncture wound with iodine-based scrub or Hibiclens – try to make puncture opening large enough for drainage – finally paint opening and into puncture as far as possible with tincture of iodine – keep wound open while drainage taking place – apply hot foments to relieve pain and aid healing.

Many puncture wounds unnoticed – if infection or dirty bodies present – abscess probably forms. Contact your veterinarian who will provide drainage, antibiotics and anti-tetanus vaccine – necessary precautions for puncture wounds.

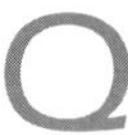

# QUEENSLAND ITCH

This disease has been recognised for years as a skin allergy. It is seasonal, occurring during the hot humid months, and the highest incidence is along the coast. It is not contagious and only hypersensitive horses show signs of it. A closely similar condition occurring in Britain, Ireland and elsewhere is known as Sweet Itch.

SIGNS
Itching, rubbing and biting – hair loss – abrasion of skin – mainly in areas of ears, mane, withers and tail – skin in longstanding cases becomes thickened, wrinkled and discoloured, with sparse hair cover.

CAUSE
Due to bites of a species of sandfly (biting midge).

TREATMENT
Sandflies most prevalent from 4 pm to early hours of evening – prevent with insect-proof stables – by rugging and hooding during these hours of the day – spraying with insecticidal solutions offers some protection.

Contact your veterinary surgeon for treatment of allergic skin reaction in some cases and for secondary infection of broken skin, caused by rubbing and biting.

# QUITTOR

Quittor is a chronic, purulent inflammation of the lateral cartilage in the hoof. It is characterised by discharge from the coronary band.

SIGNS
Redness, swelling, heat and pain in region of heel and associated coronary band – discharge from small openings or cracks around coronary band – dry up and erupt again – fluctuating lameness associated with build-up of discharge.

CAUSES
Injury near or on coronary band causing damage to cartilage and soft tissues in area of heel – a foreign body penetrating through sole in region of heel – over-reaching (see page 247).

TREATMENT
Contact your veterinary surgeon who will administer appropriate antibiotics and tetanus injections – treatment may not prove effective and complete surgical removal of diseased cartilage may be necessary – even this treatment may not effect cure.

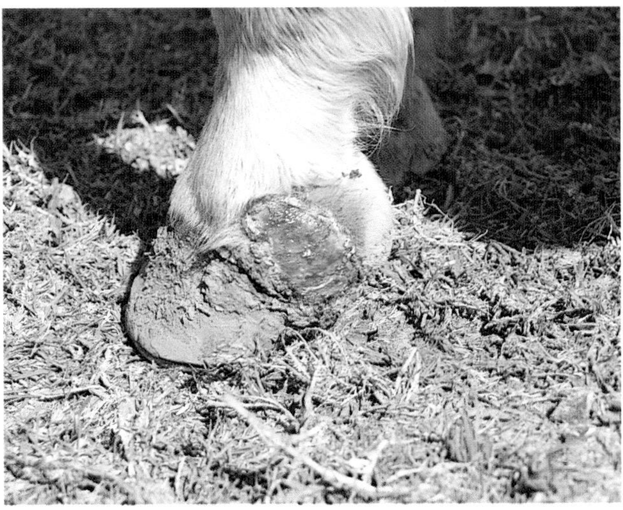

Quittor: discharging wound at the coronary band

# R

## RABIES

Rabies is a notifiable disease worldwide. It is not found in Australia.

SIGNS
Found in Europe and US – early signs: drooling of saliva – spastic lip movement – hyperexcitable – leading to depression and not eating. Rare cases become aggressive (biting and kicking). Paralysis develops – first affecting the ability to swallow and vocal cords (altered whinny) – then spreads to hindquarters with collapse and death in 2–7 days after initial signs.

CAUSE
Virus usually transmitted by bite of an infected animal – e.g. fox, skunk, raccoon, bats – saliva is highly infectious.

TREATMENT
Call your veterinarian who will contact the appropriate government authority – rabies is invariably fatal – isolate horse from other animals and people – in areas where rabies is known, protection of horse by vaccination is very effective.

## RAIN SCALD

Some horses, when exposed to the environment without shelter or protection, develop a skin irritation known as rain scald.

SIGNS
Hair on back and croup mats with inflammatory fluid that oozes from skin – some clumps of matted hair fall out – others, if peeled off, leave raw, bleeding surface.

CAUSE
Long periods of rain cause an irritation of skin on back and croup, which are flat and bear the brunt of rain as it falls.

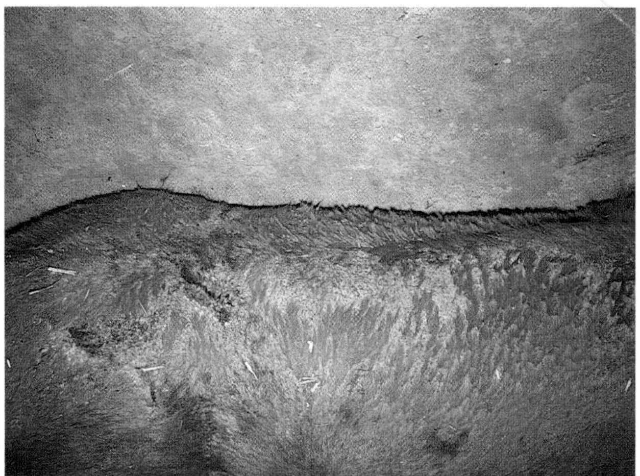

*Rain scald along the back*

TREATMENT
Provide some form of protection from elements such as stable, shelter shed, trees or rug – wash affected areas with warm water and anti-bacterial soap – gently lift any loose hair and scabs with your fingertips – dry thoroughly – groom gently and cautiously in affected areas with soft body brush – apply lanolin to exposed skin to keep it moist and supple.

# RECTO-VAGINAL FISTULA

If the tear known as a recto-vaginal fistula is not attended to, the mare is usually rendered infertile and subject to infection.

SIGNS
Tear through vaginal wall into rectum – occurs in foaling – observed without hindrance if mare's tail lifted out of way to expose anus and vulva – pulling lips of vulva apart reveals extent of tear.

CAUSES
Feet of foal pushed upwards towards rectum by mare's contractions – indicated in second stage of labour by excessive bulging of anus – eventually feet tear recto-vaginal wall if not directed downward to vaginal opening.

TREATMENT
Surgical repair by veterinary surgeon.

# RECURRENT UVEITIS (Periodic Ophthalmia)

This is the most common condition occurring inside the eyeball of horses.

SIGNS
Tears running down cheeks – sensitivity to light – closing of eyelids – conjunctivitis – pus may be in anterior chamber – sometimes inability of pupil to dilate. Generally affects horses 3–7 years of age – may clear up or improve, then recur 3–12 months later – may affect one or both eyes.

CAUSE
Infection or immune mediated disease.

TREATMENT
Call your veterinarian to make definite diagnosis – he will instil eye drops (atropine) to dilate pupil and inject a long-acting corticosteroid under conjunctiva in conjunction with antibiotic corticosteroid eye ointment. Response to treatment very good though condition likely to recur.

# RINGBONE

Ringbone is a bony swelling below the fetlock, usually located near the upper or lower joint of the pastern. A bony swelling near the upper joint is generally obvious to the naked eye and the average horseman thinks of it as the only kind of ringbone. In fact, there are two kinds. That just described is known as high ringbone; the other is called low ringbone, as it is near the lower joint of the pastern, which is encased by the hoof wall. Unless the bony swelling known as low ringbone is large enough to distend the coronary band, it cannot be seen. If the joint surface is not involved, the horse may lead a useful life, even though the bony swelling may persist.

SIGNS
If ringbone caused by injury and seen in early stages, there will be evidence of heat, swelling, pain on pressure, lameness. Ringbone resulting from poor conformation may develop slowly over long period – many such cases not diagnosed until horse shows signs of lameness – closer examination reveals bony swelling – varying in size – seen and felt on pastern.

CAUSES
Condition not inherited but conformation that predisposes horse to ringbone is inherited. Short or long upright pasterns increase concussion impact on the bone – causes inflammatory reaction on its surface – stimulates a bony growth or swelling.

Base-wide, base-narrow, toe-in and toe-out conformation predispose one side of pastern or the other to excessive strain – in turn causes ligament and joint capsule strain or tearing – sets up inflammation where ligaments or capsule are attached to bone – subsequently stimulates new bone growth.

Injury such as a kick or blow to pastern can trigger off ringbone condition. Diet low in calcium and high in phosphorus can also be predisposing cause.

TREATMENT

Seek veterinary advice – in meantime immobilise affected limb with firm pressure bandage from hoof to just below the knee. Stop all exercise and minimise movement by confining horse to stable. Cold hosing and antiphlogistine poultices will help to reduce inflammation.

With aid of X-ray, the veterinarian will vary treatment according to position, size and nature of the ringbone. Treatment ranges from radiation therapy to administering anti-inflammatory agents.

Check the affected horse's diet and correct any calcium–phosphorus imbalance.

# RINGWORM

Ringworm is a highly contagious fungal infection which may be spread by more than one type of fungus.

SIGNS

Lesions begin as circular areas of raised hair 1–3 cm in diameter – hair becomes brittle – falls out about 10 days after infection – circular clumps of hair can be plucked out – leave moist, circular, hairless lesions – sometimes dotted with a few spots of blood. Common sites of infection are head, girth and shoulders – in some cases, site is more generalised.

CAUSES

Ringworm may be spread by man – use of contaminated boots, girths, rugs, other tack and grooming gear – poor management in recognition and treatment of the infection.

Direct contact is also a cause – one infected horse infects another where body contact is possible – disease may also be spread by indirect contact – infected horse rubs against fence, depositing fungi in loose hair that can infect healthy horse if it rubs in same place.

Flies, mosquitoes and other biting insects can be responsible for spread of ringworm.

TREATMENT

Horse with ringworm usually regarded as contagious for 3 weeks from time of infection – thoroughly wash infected horse daily for

3–4 minutes in iodine-based scrub – gently lift and remove any loose scab or crust when washing – these, and any loose hair, should be collected and burned – after washing, dab hairless areas with tincture of iodine.

Isolate horse from any other non-infected horses – do not use on any healthy horse the tack or grooming gear used on infected horse – wipe tack and soak grooming gear in 0.3% Halamid solution.

If hairless areas are increasing in size or number, contact your veterinary surgeon – hair regrowth may take a month or more after successful treatment.

# ROARING (Laryngeal Hemiplegia)

## SIGNS

A peculiar noise, ranging from a whistle to a roar, that some horses make when they breathe in (inspiration) – most horses only show signs of the noise when galloping fully extended – a minority show signs even at rest.

Horse's ability to perform in events where there is stress on respiratory system is adversely affected – most often occurs in horse 16 hands or more in height and aged 3–7 years – rare in ponies.

## CAUSES

Primary cause is degeneration of nerve supplying muscles of larynx – it is known, however, that roaring is hereditary – size of horse and its conformation are inherited characteristics that can be causal factors in nerve degeneration – respiratory viruses, infections and heavy exercise can also cause roaring.

One theory is that lengthy periods of swimming cause horse to extend neck, thus stretching nerves and causing degeneration.

## TREATMENT

Success of treatment depends on accuracy of diagnosis – can only be made by a veterinary surgeon after giving horse a thorough clinical examination – includes passing up each nostril an instrument known as a rhinolaryngoscope and examining the larynx in detail.

Latest surgical technique is to pull back collapsed laryngeal cartilage and secure it permanently in its normal position by use of a prosthesis. This technique has 80–90% success rate, reducing noise level to normal at all paces.

# RUPTURED BLADDER (foal)

SIGNS
Foal shows signs of depression 12–24 hours after birth – strains repeatedly to urinate – very little or no urine passed – straining can be similar in constipated foal – do not confuse.

CAUSES
May be due to pressure on full bladder at time of foaling – or to incomplete closure of bladder during development in uterus.

TREATMENT
Contact veterinarian immediately – ruptured bladder has to be repaired surgically – success of operation depends on speed of recognition, diagnosis and surgery.

# S

## SADDLE SORE – GIRTH GALL

These sores develop because of excessive pressure and/or frictional rub from saddle or girth.

SIGNS
Hair is rubbed off and skin broken on side of withers or under girth – result of constant pressure or rubbing – often leaves raw, bleeding sores – vary in size – slow to heal.

CAUSES
Pressure brought about by an ill-fitting saddle, such as one with shallow gullet used on horse with high, narrow wither. Wrong technique may be used in saddling horse – signs are that hair is turned back rather than lying flat and smooth – saddle cloth is wrinkled – skin under girth is wrinkled – all lead to pressure and/or rubbing.

TREATMENT
Rest the horse from saddle and girth – if horse needs exercise to maintain fitness, lunge and swim it. Check saddle and girth in relation to shape of horse and technique of saddling.

Apply zinc cream to sores twice a day until they show signs of drying and healing – if sores swollen, hot, oozing and painful, contact your veterinary surgeon. Fistulous withers may develop because of an untreated, infected saddle sore on withers (see fistulous withers, page 203).

## SARCOID

Sarcoid is a skin tumour. They have not been known to spread to internal organs, but a veterinary surgeon should be consulted because of their resistance to treatment or tendency to recur.

SIGNS
Usually located on head, shoulders or lower limbs. One or several wart-like growths – vary in size from 1–10 cm in diameter – thick, crusty surface – or may be raw, ulcerated, fleshy surface that bleeds freely when touched.

## CAUSE

Virus is suspected as cause of sarcoids in horses – may gain entry into skin that has been abraded by rubbing or trauma.

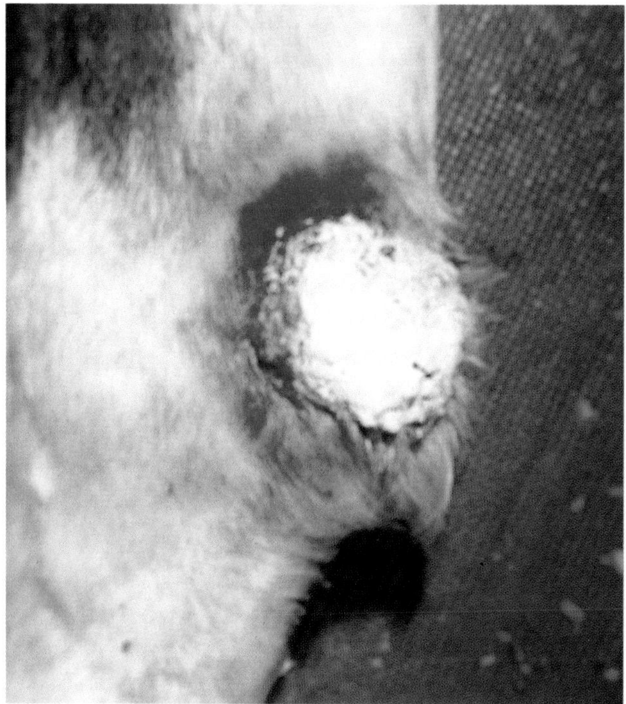

Sarcoid treated by cryosurgery (freezing)

## TREATMENT

If sarcoid small (1 cm), paint with Podophyllin, taking care not to get it on normal skin as severe burning will follow. Often when sarcoid painted with Podophyllin, it runs off surface of sarcoid onto skin. As preventive measure, smear vaseline on skin around the sarcoid before painting – continue applying paint until sarcoid has been burned back to skin level. If sarcoid recurs, or is larger than 1 cm, contact your veterinarian – he may cauterise or surgically excise the lesion. Even after surgical excision, sarcoid can recur. Only answer is further surgical excision, followed by radiation treatment.

# SARCOPTIC MANGE (Scabies)

SIGNS
Severe irritation – initially on head and neck – extending to other parts of body – does not involve mane, tail or lower limbs. Small nodules form – often with scab on top – hair loss – moth-eaten appearance – skin becomes thickened – forms into folds – weight loss.

Itchy red spots form on inside of forearms and exposed skin of stablehands having close contact with horse.

CAUSE
Sarcoptes mange mite burrows into skin of head, shoulders and neck causing intense irritation – can occur in irregular patches all over skin.

TREATMENT
Definite diagnosis made by veterinarian scraping skin deeply and examining it under microscope – dip, rinse, spray with organophosphorus compound such as Bayer Asuntol – treat all horses that have had contact though they may show no signs. Check bedding, tack, loose hair, grooming equipment and stables.

# SEEDY TOE

SIGNS
Separation of wall from sole at the toe – leaves a pocket or cavity running under wall – if hoof wall is tapped, it emits hollow sound – when shoe is removed and sole is pared back at toe, a hollow cavity is visible – often filled with black, foul-smelling, greasy, decaying hoof – horse may or may not be lame.

CAUSES
Chronic founder – poor hoof trimming and shoeing – foreign body such as a small stone wedging between wall and sole at toe.

TREATMENT
With hoof knife, cut away dead, black horn lining cavity until you reach good healthy horn – paint inside of cavity daily for 7 days with solution containing 10% formalin. Most cases that recur do so because dead horn has not been cut out completely. If seedy toe is of a deep nature, call your veterinarian, as antibiotics and tetanus injection may be indicated.

# SEPTICAEMIA (Blood Poisoning)

Septicaemia is the circulation of bacteria in large numbers in the bloodstream.

SIGNS
Foal depressed – shows weakness – fails to suckle – breathes rapidly – lies down – harsh coat – temperature initially high then falls and becomes sub-normal as foal deteriorates – foal may die suddenly.

CAUSES
Bacteria can enter foal's bloodstream in a number of ways – bacteria can pass from mare's bloodstream across placenta to foal's bloodstream – stump of umbilical cord after birth is a common route of infection – skin wounds, however slight, provide a means for penetration of bacteria – contaminated food, milk, or foreign bodies, if taken into mouth and swallowed, are a source of infection – foal sniffing around, particularly on ground, can inhale bacteria.

TREATMENT
Keep foal warm, quiet and confined – contact your veterinarian – he will administer antibiotics and fluids intravenously (to counteract shock and dehydration) – a blood sample will be taken to culture and identify the bacterium and to do a sensitivity test to identify the antibiotic that is most effective against that particular bacterium.

Many infections in foals can be prevented by stud masters:

- avoiding overuse of their foaling yard;
- taking care to see mare and foal are kept in a clean environment;
- swabbing foal's umbilical cord liberally with tincture of iodine immediately it is born;
- checking that the foal has had its colostrum from the mare shortly after birth.

# SESAMOIDITIS

Sesamoiditis is inflammation of the two sesamoid bones at the back of the fetlock joint. They act as pulleys for the flexor tendons that pass over them and provide attachment for the suspensory ligament.

SIGNS
Swelling at back of fetlock – lameness – pain on application of

pressure to sesamoid bones and on bending fetlock joint – in some cases only sign is horse stepping short.

CAUSES
Sesamoid bones are subject to pulling effect from ligaments attached to them – constant pulling can aggravate the surface of the bones – sets up inflammation – can be further aggravated by conformational faults such as long, sloping pasterns or by activities such as racing, jumping and hunting.

TREATMENT
Rest and immobilisation are desirable – pressure bandage should be applied from just below knee to top of hoof. Paint back of fetlock joint with cooling lotion. Trimming and rasping hoof to shorten toe and fitting shoe with raised heel tapering down to a rolled toe will help relieve strain on sesamoid bones.

Consult your veterinary surgeon – with aid of X-ray he may vary treatment – may involve anti-inflammatory agents, 6 months rest or radiation therapy.

# SHIN SORENESS

Shin soreness is common among young thoroughbreds. The forelimb is the usual site – occurrence in the hind limb is comparatively rare. The condition is caused by excessive demands on the horse to exert itself physically. Shin soreness (bucked shins or metacarpal periostitis) results from a tearing of the periosteum (the membrane covering the bone) along the front of the metacarpal (cannon) bone. Some trainers think shin soreness is inevitable but this idea is quite false. Many cases can be avoided by paying attention to diet, foot trimming, shoeing, track surface and training methods.

SIGNS
Swelling on front of cannon bone warm to touch – painful when pressure exerted. Lameness increases with exercise – stride will be characterised by a short anterior phase – if only one limb is involved, horse will tend to rest it – if both limbs involved horse will shift its weight from one to the other.

CAUSES
Concussion probably most frequent cause, particularly in young horses. Common digital extensor tendon runs across front of cannon bone, very loosely tied down to it by fibrous bands – periosteal attachment to the bone in young horses is immature – more readily pulled away from the bone – causes inflammation. Injuries to periosteum from direct trauma may also produce sore shins. Shin soreness in one leg only, or in mature horses, is often

caused by trauma, such as hitting cannon bone on yard rail or feed tin.

Small saucer-like and hairline fractures can be underlying causes of shin soreness – generally show severe inflammation, localised to small area on front surface of cannon bone – severe cases of shin soreness should be X-rayed to eliminate possibility of such fractures.

### TREATMENT

Rest essential for complete recovery – use of counter-irritants, anti-inflammatory drugs, X-ray therapy and cobalt 60 are of real value. Selection of treatment depends on severity of case and on actual cause of shin soreness.

# SIDEBONE

Calcification (formation of bone) of the cartilages attached to the wing of the pedal bone is known as sidebone, a condition usually found in heavy breeds. It is not common in thoroughbreds.

### SIGNS

May or may not be lame – lameness may be evident when horse turns – heat and pain over heels of foot – usually occurs in forefeet – may be visible bulging of coronary band over the quarters of hoof – pressing the area reveals cartilages have lost elasticity because they are calcified. Diagnosis of sidebone is confirmed by X-ray.

### CAUSES

Repeated concussion of hoof causing inflammation of pedal bone and associated lateral cartilages – poor conformation (toe-in and toe-out) – poor trimming and shoeing over a lengthy period, increasing concussion of the hoof.

### TREATMENT

Many horses have sidebone without any sign of lameness – if lameness due to sidebone and confirmed by your veterinarian he can administer anti-inflammatory agents orally or by injection to reduce inflammation and pain – rest is recommended – if X-ray reveals small fragment of sidebone is broken off, it can be removed surgically – recovery is favourable.

# SINUSITIS

Sinusitis is not uncommon, partly because of the large sinus cavities in the horse's head (frontal and maxillary sinuses).

SIGNS

Nasal discharge from one nostril thick and foul smelling, possibly streaked with blood – may be swelling above or below eye – may be discharge from eye – if sinus full of pus it emits dull sound when tapped.

CAUSES

Infection – trauma – infected root of a tooth – tumour.

TREATMENT

Feed horse from ground to facilitate better drainage – thorough, frequent cleaning of feed bin and water container – contact your veterinarian who will diagnose cause of the sinusitis – swab culture and X-rays – will treat horse with antibiotics and/or surgery. To trephine the sinus is to make large hole to allow irrigation with antibiotic solutions.

# SOFT PALATE DISPLACEMENT

The soft palate in the horse is long and this is the reason why the horse breathes through its nose and not its mouth. The soft palate normally lies below the opening (epiglottis) of the windpipe – when displaced it lies over the opening of the windpipe, obstructing the airflow.

SIGNS

Noise during strenuous exercise, e.g. extended gallop – often towards end of race – horse makes a loud choking noise associated with inspiration (breathing in) and expiration (breathing out) – when it occurs horse will almost stop.

CAUSE

Unknown, but may be related to muscles which control position of larynx.

TREATMENT

Call your veterinarian to confirm diagnosis by examination with an endoscope – instrument to look up nasal passages at soft palate and associated structures – often, at rest, soft palate is in its normal position – diagnosis is usually made on history, track inspection, endoscope examination and elimination of other respiratory problems.

Use of a tongue tie or straight bit will stop displacement of soft palate – otherwise surgical correction indicated if this conservative approach fails.

# SPLINTS

Splints, a condition mainly of young horses, most often affects the forelimbs. It is associated with hard training, poor conformation, malnutrition and immaturity. This disease is most commonly found on the medial (inside) aspect of the limb between the 2nd and 3rd metacarpal bones, because of the shape of the proximal ends of the bones and the fact that the second metacarpal normally bears more weight. It is less common on the lateral (outer) side between the 3rd and 4th metacarpal bones. Occasionally, it occurs among 3- and 4-year-olds.

## SIGNS

May occur anywhere along length of splint bone – more common at its junction with third metacarpal bone – heat, pain and swelling in affected area. Splint formation near knee may cause arthritis to develop – excessive bone growth may put pressure on suspensory ligament and cause chronic lameness – some cases of splints may never cause lameness.

After original inflammation subsides, enlargement usually becomes smaller but firmer as result of ossification at site of swelling. In early stages greatest bulk of swelling is fibrous tissue – this normally resolves to a much smaller size – reduction in swelling usually due to decrease in amount of fibrous tissue, not to decrease in size of actual bone formation.

Fracture of splint bone commonly confused with splints – whenever one suspects splint bone fracture X-rays should be taken by veterinary surgeon.

## CAUSES

Concussion that results from working on hard surfaces may cause disturbance to fibrous interosseous ligament between 2nd and 3rd or 3rd and 4th metacarpal bones – this may cause irritation of periosteum, which could lead to periostitis and new bone growth, a condition commonly referred to as splints.

Splints may also be produced by trauma resulting from blows to outside of limb or from interference to inner side – any trauma induced by slipping, running, jumping or falling may be enough to disturb interosseous ligament before it becomes ossified.

Faulty conformation may cause splints by placing abnormal stresses on interosseous ligaments.

Deficiencies of calcium, phosphorus, vitamin A or vitamin D in horse's diet may also predispose it to splints.

## TREATMENT

Varies according to size, position and nature of splint – can range from anti-inflammatory preparations to surgical removal and cobalt treatment. In every case, important to analyse horse's diet and blood to determine if deficiencies exist that predispose horse to the condition. Prognosis favourable in all cases except where bony growth is large and encroaches on suspensory ligament and/or carpal knee joint.

# SPONDYLITIS

Spondylitis is inflammation of the vertebrae, the bones that make up the spinal column. The most common site of inflammation is the lumbar area, between the back and the croup. In some horses, primarily hunters, there is involvement of the sacroiliac joint, located where the spine joins the pelvis. Inflammation of the vertebrae over a long period often produces spur formations on the under edge of the vertebrae. These spurs grow towards each other, finally joining together to form a bridge (a condition called ankylosing spondylitis). Once the vertebrae have ankylosed there is a reduction of movement or flexibility in the back, accompanied by a reduction in pain.

When a horse is sensitive to touch along its back or tends to half-squat when running water is sprayed on its back, some trainers wrongly say that it has kidney trouble. This is rare in horses and the cause of pain is much more likely to be spondylitis. The condition is fairly common in racing horses, both thoroughbreds and standard breds.

## SIGNS

If enough pressure applied to back of any horse it will flinch and tend to squat – some horses will flinch and squat sometimes to point of sitting like a dog, when only light pressure from tip of a pen is run down either side of spine – when saddled up for riding some horses will straighten back and half squat or arch back as if they are going to buck.

Twitching of tail, restlessness, laying back ears, and inability to stand still indicate back pain.

Some horses, when rider mounts, half squat and often walk off in that position for half a dozen paces before straightening up – during exercise the horse may feel unco-ordinated in hind-quarters or may not be able to stretch out properly.

After work when horse hosed down, running water from hose played onto its back may make it squat – when grooming horse, effect of brush on its back may also cause it to squat – keep in mind that some horses with sensitive skin do not like to be groomed.

## CAUSES

Positioning of saddle too far back – often occurs with heavy riders – bucking and pigrooting can also cause spondylitis – head check on standard breds may be too short, horse may carry its head high thereby indirectly putting pressure on lower back – too much stress may be placed on the back of a hunter.

When horse galloping and front legs are extended or stretched well forward, there is a concave effect on lower spine – as front and hind limbs come together, lower spine forms an arch or convexity – as horse gallops, shape of lower spine changes constantly from concave to convex – action causes inflammation of surface of involved vertebrae in spine.

TREATMENT
Rest offers immediate relief – in many cases symptoms recur on return to work – alternative to rest is to give affected horse a different training program with less pressure or weight on back.

Make sure saddle fits horse properly and is well forward, with plenty of padding underneath – if horse being prepared for racing, use a lightweight work rider and instruct him to ride with his weight well forward.

Try to curb any bucking, pigrooting or kicking up of hind legs.

Paint muscles on both sides of spinal column with cooling lotion and consult your veterinary surgeon about using an anti-inflammatory agent.

# STALL WALKING

This vice is closely related to weaving.

SIGNS
Horse constantly walks in circles around stable – often wears deep track in earthen floor – causes fatigue and strain on legs.

CAUSE
Bored and nervous.

TREATMENT
Place horse in yard or paddock with placid companion. Tying up horse or placing objects, e.g. bales of straw, in stable help prevent stall walking.

# STRANGLES

Strangles is a highly contagious acute disease of young horses, characterised by abscess formation, especially in the submaxillary glands (under the jaw), and inflammation of the upper respiratory tract with nasal discharge.

SIGNS
First symptoms are loss of appetite followed by slight cough. Within few days, bilateral nasal discharge develops which becomes copious. Lymph nodes of head and neck may become inflamed and swollen, those under jaw being first affected. If sinusitis or inflammation of guttural pouches develops, surgical attention may be necessary. Laryngitis may develop and lead to laryngeal hemiplegia (broken wind), if horse is being exercised.

Strangles can spread to other parts of the body and localise in areas such as lungs. It if does, it is referred to as 'bastard strangles'.

CAUSES
Organism causing strangles is bacterium *Streptococcus equi*, which can be found in pus discharge from nose or from abscesses under jaw. The bacteria in the pus are fairly resistant to the environment – their presence in paddocks, feed or water troughs is a source of infection – gain entry into body by ingestion or inhalation. Outbreaks of strangles occur most commonly when large numbers of horses are kept together – many outbreaks thought to be initiated by a carrier, i.e. an infected horse which appears normal.

TREATMENT
Call your veterinarian – he will treat horse with antibiotics and surgically attend to any abscesses if drainage required. While waiting for veterinarian to arrive – isolate horse from any others – provide good general nursing – early treatment often brings about a quick cure – prevents spread of disease to other parts of body.

Vaccination is used extensively in treatment of strangles – it was developed because recovery from strangles usually accompanied by lasting immunity. Old vaccines caused a tissue reaction ranging from local soreness to large painful swelling – more recent vaccine has minimal side effects – initial course involves 3 vaccinations given 2 weeks apart – effective immunity is reached 2 weeks after last vaccination.

# STRINGHALT

Stringhalt is observed when the horse is in motion. One or both hind limbs are alternately raised with a high-stepping, jerky, almost spastic type of movement. The condition can be mistaken for a more common one in which the kneecap becomes fixed, locking the leg (see locking of stifle on page 237).

SIGNS
When horse moves or turns, hind limbs are raised alternately with sudden high action as if horse were reacting to sharp pain in foot. When horse is motionless, there is no evident sign of disease.

CAUSES
Condition is uncommon – true cause is not known, although diseases of nervous system are implicated – in Australia, horses

grazing on pastures containing dandelion weed may develop stringhalt.

TREATMENT
Check pasture for dandelion weed – move horse to different paddock – if no improvement, call your veterinarian, who may recommend surgical removal of a section of tendon that crosses outside of hock.

# SUMMER SORES (Habronema Infestation)

This is a seasonal skin condition which can reach epidemic proportions in summer.

SIGNS
Fleshy tissue develops from wound or moist region such as eye, penis or prepuce – tends to improve naturally in winter and flare up in summer.

CAUSE
Larvae of Habronema (a parasite which lives in stomach). Flies carry Habronema larvae – feed on wounds or around moist areas such as eyes – larvae enter tissue causing fleshy tissue growth reaction.

TREATMENT
Your veterinarian can make definite diagnosis by taking tissue biopsy for pathological examination. He may treat it by injection – local application of anthelmintics to tissues – sometimes in conjunction with surgical excision.

Prevention: bandage fresh wounds – institute fly control program.

# SUNBURN

Areas around the head and back are particularly susceptible to sunburn, especially in hot regions where the sun is fierce for many days of the year.

SIGNS
Hairless, non-pigmented areas such as nose become red, swollen, and ooze serum – skin often peels – leaves raw, bleeding areas – very sensitive to touch. Along back of horse serum mats with

hair, dries, hardens and peels – after long period skin becomes dry and wrinkled, with little or no hair cover.

CAUSES
Number of sunburn cases associated with grazing on certain lush clover pastures that appear to make skin, especially the non-pigmented areas, hypersensitive to sunlight. Non-pigmented and hairless skin, e.g. on muzzle, more easily burned by hot sun.

TREATMENT
Provide shade in form of stable, shed or trees – horses that will not stand in shade in paddock should be placed in enclosed stable. Apply zinc cream to burned areas – provides barrier against sun as well as soothes skin – where skin is not peeling, sun-screen preparations are beneficial.

If horse grazing on lush clover – remove it from paddock – hand feed it with oaten hay and small quantity of grain. If skin over large area has been severely burned, contact your veterinarian.

# SUPERNUMERARY TEETH

SIGNS
Sometimes permanent incisors erupt behind temporary incisors – temporary teeth remain firmly embedded in gum – gives horse one or two extra teeth or sometimes a complete second row – food collects between teeth – sets up inflammation and infection.

CAUSE
Genetic.

TREATMENT
Your veterinarian will distinguish temporary teeth from permanent ones and extract them.

# SUSPENSORY LIGAMENT SPRAIN

The suspensory ligament starts at the back of the cannon bone, near to its top. Seven centimetres above the fetlock it divides into two branches which wrap around either side of the sesamoid bones. Sprain of the ligament usually occurs at the site of division or in one of the branches.

SIGNS

Swelling at back of cannon bone between flexor tendons and cannon bone. Horse usually not lame but will not stretch out – pain on palpation of suspensory ligament – may be swelling and pain with pressure where suspensory ligament divides into two branches about 7 cm above fetlock.

CAUSES

Over-extension of the fetlock joint – long sloping pasterns – hooves with long toe and low heel may place excess stress on suspensory ligament when horse in motion.

TREATMENT

Up to 12 months rest. Immediately after injury – cold hose – ice pack – pressure bandage – anti-inflammatory treatment by veterinarian. Surgery involving carbon fibre implants or sclerosing agents has been used with limited success.

# SWOLLEN LEGS

Swollen legs may be seen in horses in training, on a high-grain diet or confined to a small stable or yard. The swelling may be in one leg or in all four, but is more commonly seen in both hind legs. Such a condition is often referred to as 'humor' in the leg(s).

SIGNS

Swelling usually involves pastern, fetlock and either side of flexor tendons to just below knee – may be warm to touch but not painful – when pressed with finger temporary depression left in skin – indicates fluid present in tissues underneath – stiffness when moving may be evident.

CAUSES

If infection or trauma of limb(s) not obvious, lack of exercise together with high-grain diet, leading to poor circulation of both blood and lymph in lower limbs, are predisposing causes.

TREATMENT

Walking and trotting exercise morning and afternoon – hot fomentations followed by cold hosing of affected leg(s) for 10 minutes, morning and night – massage limbs – pressure bandage them to keep swelling down – laxative in form of bran mash should be given – reduce concentrates in diet – increase roughage. When horse is not in training reduce concentrates, particularly grain, in diet. Horses returning from spelling paddock should be slowly reintroduced to work and to grain in diet.

# T

## TETANUS

This disease is found throughout the world and affects all domestic animals except the cat. It is common in horses. Tetanus is a toxaemia or poisoning produced by the bacterial agent *Clostridium tetani*. It is characterised by spasmodic muscular contractions, in many cases resulting in death.

### SIGNS

Stiffness – rigidity of whole body – third eyelids partially cover the eyes – difficulty with taking food into mouth and chewing – drooling a mixture of saliva and food – general stiffness leads to convulsions and death in up to 80% of cases.

### CAUSE

*Clostridium tetani* produces a toxin or poison that affects nervous system – organism lives in soil and horse faeces (manure) – tetanus spores persist in ground for long time and are resistant to many standard disinfectants, including steam at 100°C for 30–60 minutes. Puncture wounds of hoof are not infrequently associated with development of tetanus – entry of tetanus is usually via a deep wound – even then, it may lie dormant for 4 months until conditions are suitable for tetanus spores to multiply and produce toxin.

### TREATMENT

Call your veterinarian immediately. However, supportive therapy by the owner can be almost as important as veterinary treatment.

Place horse in a quiet, dark stall, with a deep bed of straw – if possible, do not handle – remove any objects that could cause injury – place feed bins and water containers at such a height that the horse does not have to bend down – feed it bran mashes (see page 45) to minimise necessity to chew as well as to prevent constipation.

Vaccination with tetanus toxoid extremely important for all horses – active immunity takes 14 days to develop – horse must be vaccinated before exposure to infection – initial course usually consists of two doses given about 4 weeks apart. Injection of tetanus toxoid often produces swelling in muscle at site of injection – disappears in about 4 days – not true that vaccination will adversely affect horse's performance for rest of its life.

Foals should be vaccinated at 3–4 months of age – mares in last month of pregnancy so that temporary immunity will be passed onto foal – outside mares on arrival at stud should have booster vaccination – all horses should have yearly booster because of frequency of cuts, nail pricks, castration wounds, foaling lacerations and general trauma.

If horse has suffered a wound in which tetanus infection likely, your veterinary surgeon can administer an antitoxin that will give immediate protection and afford temporary immunity for about 2 weeks. Any person involved with horses should consult their doctor about tetanus vaccination.

# THOROUGH PIN

This condition is a swelling of the tendon sheath near the point of the hock. Distension is usually evident on both sides of the hock.

SIGNS
Swelling under skin in tendon sheath above point of hock – usually evident on both sides – swelling soft and mobile – more common in young horses.

CAUSE
Hard work, especially in young immature horses.

TREATMENT
Rest – cold hosing – painting with a cooling lotion. Drainage by veterinarian sometimes necessary.

# THRUSH

Thrush is an infection located in the grooves on either side of the frog. Sometimes the frog itself is involved.

SIGNS
Foul-smelling, black, tarry discharge can be seen in grooves on either side of frog – horse may be lame if sensitive tissues in depths of grooves are involved.

CAUSES
Predisposing causes that provide breeding ground for infection are poor hoof care – particularly lack of attention to daily cleaning and hoof trimming at time of shoeing – damp, dirty stable

conditions where horse stands in bedding soaked with urine and manure – poorly drained yards, with horse standing for lengthy periods in mud or in damp, dirty places.

TREATMENT
Trim away any excess or infected frog – clean out discharge from grooves – if sensitive tissues involved, horse will flinch or pull foot away when you dig deeply into grooves. Paint sole, including depths of grooves, with solution of 10% formalin – be careful not to bring skin into contact with formalin – severe burning may result. Repeat treatment daily until condition has cleared up completely.

Contact your veterinary surgeon, as antibiotics and tetanus injections may be indicated.

Cleanliness is keynote to prevention of thrush. Daily hoof and stable cleaning are thus important – when trimming and shoeing horse, it is essential to maintain frog contact with ground – if this not possible, a bar shoe should be fitted to exert pressure on frog.

# THYROID GLAND ENLARGEMENT

The thyroid gland is located on either side of the upper section of the windpipe, but is only obvious when enlarged. It is not uncommon to find one or both sides of the thyroid gland enlarged in horses in training.

SIGNS
Swelling on upper section of windpipe – on one or both sides – firm, mobile, oval-shaped, 4–7 cm across – loss of condition – weakness – decreased libido – obesity.

CAUSES
Deficiency in iodine. Iodine-deficient areas occur in Australia, Britain, North and South America and Europe. Horses grazing on natural pasture and drinking water in these areas may suffer from iodine deficiency. Those on high calcium or linseed meal diets cannot absorb or utilise iodine efficiently.

TREATMENT
Commercially prepared iodised salt or mineral supplement containing iodine fed to horse can bring about quick remission of signs of iodine deficiency – prolonged dosing or overdosing with iodine can produce serious illness – do not use it indiscriminately but consult your veterinarian for advice.

# TUMORAL CALCINOSIS

SIGNS
Round, hard, immobile swelling(s) – 4–14 cm in diameter on outside of leg below stifle – usually first noticed in weanlings and yearlings – as a rule, no lameness.

CAUSE
Unknown.

TREATMENT
Best left untreated – blemish rather than hindrance – can usually be removed surgically.

# TUMOUR

Tumours of the nasal cavity and sinuses are not uncommon in the horse.

SIGNS
Clear or purulent mucus, sometimes tinged with blood, from one nostril – abnormal sound coming from nostril especially when horse worked – may be no movement of air in or out of nostril – detected by placing hand over it – may be swelling of one side of nasal cavity in association with watery and bulging eye.

CAUSE
Unknown.

TREATMENT
Contact your veterinarian who can confirm diagnosis with endoscope and X-ray examination. Polyps may be successfully removed – many tumours cannot be successfully treated with either surgery or radiation therapy.

# TYING-UP

Tying-up is a less severe form of azoturia (see page 160).

SIGNS
During or after work horse steps short in hind limbs, giving appearance of stiffness – only sign may be that horse will not stretch out during training or when competing – horses with these signs normally on high-grain diet and only show signs when worked after a day or more of rest.

## CAUSES

Physiology of tying-up not yet fully understood. Horses worked at irregular intervals and fed high-grain diets are most susceptible to tying-up.

Ingested grain converted to glycogen, which is stored in muscles and elsewhere – if horse rested for 1–2 days while on a high-grain diet, large quantities of glycogen are stored in muscles – glycogen is used by muscles as a source of energy when work is being done – waste product from chemical change that takes place is lactic acid – if large volume of glycogen is stored, a large volume of lactic acid is produced when horse exercises – if lactic acid cannot be expelled from muscle tissue, it damages fibres, causing condition known as tying-up.

Some horses not on high-grain diets tie up because they are hypersensitive to lactic acid or because their particular metabolism does not cope with it efficiently.

## TREATMENT

Call your veterinarian who can confirm the condition – by its history, clinical signs and taking a blood sample for certain serum enzyme tests – if horse has elevated serum enzyme levels, indicating muscle inflammation, days before an event it is a good idea to taper horse's training program to allow the muscle inflammation to subside – will help horse perform to best of its ability on day of event.

Sub-clinical cases are those not performing well but exhibit no other signs – a blood test is only way of diagnosing them.

Horses susceptible to frequent tying-up should have low-level grain diet – normally grain level in diet should be in proportion to amount of work done – exercise horse every day, even if it is just walking exercise – consult your veterinarian about use of vitamin E and selenium as preventive measure.

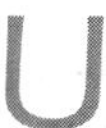

# UMBILICAL HERNIA

This is a congenital defect. Sometimes a loop of intestine passing through an opening in the muscular wall becomes twisted. It strangles itself and cuts off the blood supply to it in that section. Emergency surgery is necessary to save the foal's life.

SIGNS
Swelling in region of navel – may be up to 5 cm in diameter.

CAUSES
Fatty tissue or intestine passes through hole in muscle group and presses against skin of abdominal wall.

TREATMENT
Many small umbilical hernias close up and disappear over period of 12 months – wise to ask veterinary surgeon to evaluate hernia and decide if surgery is necessary.

# UNDERSHOT JAW

This condition is commonly known as parrot mouth.

SIGNS
Upper and lower incisors do not meet because lower jaw is too short.

CAUSE
Possibly genetic.

TREATMENT
Nil – if lower incisors tend to push up into hard palate they should be filed and checked every 3 months.

# V

## VERMINOUS ANEURYSM

An aneurysm is a localised thickening of the wall of an artery, causing restriction of the blood flow. It results from disease or injury.

SIGNS
Horse may be exercised for lengthy periods before lameness evident in hind limbs – or severe lameness may be evident immediately after exercise begins – affected hind leg will be cool to touch – shows little or no sign of sweating – rest of body may sweat profusely. Horse shows signs of pain and anxiety – lameness disappears with rest.

CAUSE
Verminous aneurysm is most common form of aneurysm found in horse. Larvae of red worm, *Strongylus vulgaris*, migrate into muscular walls of arteries – particularly posterior aorta or iliac arteries supplying hind limbs – larvae set up inflammation – fibrous swelling develops – over time fibrous swelling reduces diameter of lumen of artery – restricts blood flow to hind limbs – arterial wall may become so thickened that blood supply is cut off.

TREATMENT
Once a verminous aneurysm develops, no known treatment will cause it to regress – only the symptoms caused by aneurysm can be treated – routine and correct worming procedures, especially with young horses, cannot be overemphasised in preventing development of verminous aneurysm.

# VICES (Kicking; Striking; Biting; Rearing; Pulling Back)

SIGNS
Kicking, e.g. stable doors and tailgates of floats – rearing with flailing legs – striking – turning round, presenting hindquarters, one leg raised as warning – pulling back – laying back ears, extending neck, showing teeth ready to bite.

CAUSES
Vicious – nervous – excitable – stubborn – temperamental – poor training.

TREATMENT
Consider your personal approach to horse – its background – seek help from professional handler – horses that habitually kick, rear, bite, etc, are undesirable.

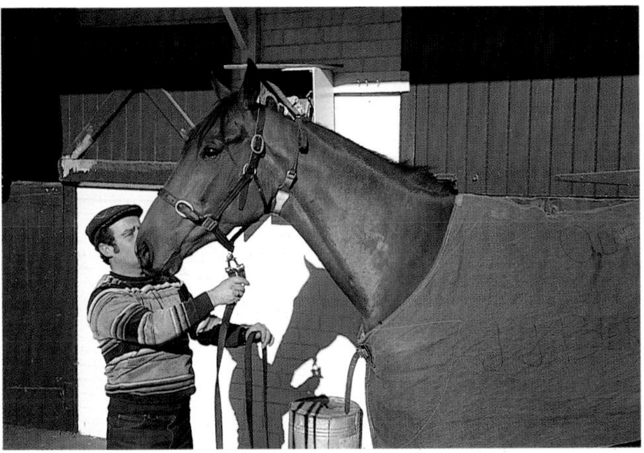

Crib biting (see p. 189) is a vice caused by boredom. This special strap, fitted tightly round the neck, can be effective in preventing it.

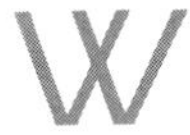

# WARTS

Warts usually occur around the heads of young horses up to 3 years old. They can vary in number from a few to hundreds.

SIGNS
Lumps varying in size from 2 mm to 2 cm – common sites are nose, lips, eyelids and cheeks – colour from pink to grey – have raised, rough, horny surface.

CAUSE
Virus can be transmitted from one horse to another, probably gaining entry through cut or abrasion in skin – biting flies may be involved in spread.

TREATMENT
Condition self-limiting, usually regressing within 3 months. Sometimes warts can be broken by rubbing, they bleed and are susceptible to fly strike – in these cases, crude castor oil will eradicate them – castor oil should be carefully applied to wart only, not to surrounding skin. If warts a problem – especially on horse studs – fences, stables, head collars and brushes should be thoroughly cleaned with formalin solution.

# WEAK FLEXOR TENDONS

SIGN
Foal walks on back of fetlock joint.

CAUSES
Particular cause of limb deformities difficult to isolate – may be a single one or combination of several – generally, causes may be classified as nutritional, malpositioning of foal in mare's uterus, inherited genetic abnormalities or injury.

TREATMENT
Essential to treat deformity as soon as possible to remedy it – failing that, to stabilise it. It is always wise to check nutritional

status of mare and foal – if necessary supplement their diet with vitamin and mineral supplement rich in calcium. Confine foal to stable with deep bed of straw. Some cases require a light fibreglass cast to support fetlock for few days.

# WEAVING

SIGNS
Horse swings head and neck from side to side – alternates weight on front legs with each swing – legs may be stressed and horse fatigued.

CAUSE
Nervous – highly strung – accentuated by boredom.

TREATMENT
Hang objects from roof rafters especially in doorways – alleviate boredom in same way as for crib biter (see page 189).

# WEIGHT LOSS

Many performance horses when in hard training and competing have poor appetite and weight loss leading to poor performance.

SIGNS
Horse's normal bodily condition must be taken into consideration – could be obese, well-muscled, thin or emaciated – well-muscled, thin horses are physiologically normal. Signs we are concerned with are horses losing weight associated with training, competing and poor performance.

CAUSES
Stress produces poor appetite – decrease in protein intake associated with hard work can cause weight loss – more subtle cause of weight loss can be increased amount of grain being fed horse to provide energy for hard work – grains, e.g. oats, are a poor source of protein. Hard work causes muscle fibre fatigue – if prolonged, leads to muscle fibre breakdown – puts horse in negative nitrogen balance.

TREATMENT
Serum protein levels evaluated on a blood count by your veterinarian – determine whether a high-protein feed additive such as soy bean meal, cottonseed meal or dried powdered milk is required – beware of some high-protein feeds such as linseed meal – very low in digestibility.

Certain anabolic steroids can be used – stimulate appetite, assist in efficiently converting protein in diet to muscle and other kinds of tissue – offset muscle fibre breakdown – put horse into a positive nitrogen balance.

Teeth should be examined regularly every 6 weeks – teeth problems such as sharp edges causing lacerations to inside of cheeks can cause horse to go off its feed.

Check for parasites every six weeks.

# WIND GALL

Surrounding a joint or tendon is a capsule or sheath, producing synovial fluid that acts as a lubricant. If the capsule is damaged by concussion or stretching, it produces excess synovial fluid that makes the capsule bulge to form what is known as a wind gall.

SIGNS
Soft, round, fluid-filled swelling – commonly appears on either side off and just above fetlock joint – about 2 cm in diameter – not accompanied by heat, pain or lameness – increase in size as workload increases.

CAUSES
Concussion or hard work may cause overextension or overflexion.

TREATMENT
An antiphlogistine poultice – cold compresses – drainage and injection of anti-inflammatory agent by veterinary surgeon.

True wind gall is only a blemish. If it is accompanied by lameness, heat or pain, area should be thoroughly examined for further problems.

# WOBBLER

This disease is characterised by poor co-ordination and weakness, particularly in the hindquarters. It is seen most commonly in male thoroughbreds, usually before they reach 2 years of age.

SIGNS
Poor co-ordination – wobbling – weakness – clumsiness – not wanting to lie down or roll. Condition may remain static or progress from slight wobbling to exaggerated, drunken movements, with horse crashing into objects and obstacles such as doorways.

Generally recognised in horses from 1–2 years of age when they are being broken in, educated and exercised.

## CAUSES

General opinion is that narrowing of canal formed by vertebrae (bones) in neck causes damage to spinal cord, which in turn is responsible for wobbler condition.

The disease may be inherited – occurs 5 times more frequently in males than in females – its incidence in thoroughbreds is far greater than in other breeds – heavily muscled, well-developed horses appear to be affected more often than others.

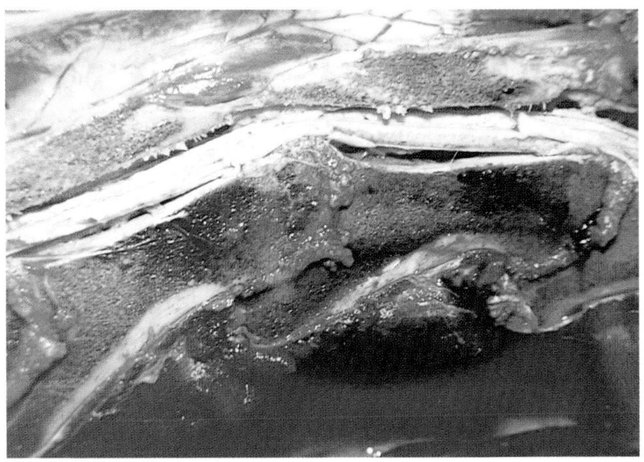

Post-mortem of a wobbler shows narrowing of the spinal canal causing compression of the spinal cord

## TREATMENT

If you suspect your horse is a wobbler, contact your veterinarian, who will conduct detailed tests and take X-rays in order to confirm or dispel your suspicions.

The author has heard of various types of people bringing about miraculous cures – in these cases, either the horses were not true wobblers to begin with or the 'permanent cure' claims are not genuine – no medication treatment has proved effective – temporary improvement has been observed in some cases after treatment. Surgery is currently being performed to stabilise affected vertebrae in neck – the long-term results of such operations are not available.

Wobblers present their owners with an unhappy situation – their usefulness, in terms of ability to perform, is severely restricted – potentially, wobblers are a source of danger – if they are so badly affected that they cannot fend for themselves in a paddock or are constantly injuring themselves, euthanasia should be considered.

# WOOD CHEWING

This vice can be costly, as horses have been known to chew through stable doors and fences.

SIGNS
Chewed timber doors, fences, stable walls – worn incisor teeth – abscesses in mouth, on lips, from splinters – colic.

CAUSES
Boredom – irritated teeth – dietary deficiency – parasites.

TREATMENT
Hay net diverts attention of horse away from this vice – capping doorways and exposed timber with metal strips and painting timber with creosote may be helpful – replacing stable doors and jambs with metal, timber rails in fences with wire, are useful deterrents.

# WOUNDS, INCISED

SIGNS
Wound edges clean cut – fairly well opposed – minimum tissue damage.

CAUSE
Sharp objects such as edge of galvanised iron used to make stables.

TREATMENT
Call veterinary surgeon to suture wound – should be stitched within 8 hours of accident – stitches removed 10–12 days later.

# INDEX